ALCOHOL AND THE FETUS

ALCOHOL AND THE FETUS

A Clinical Perspective

Henry L. Rosett, M.D.
CLINICAL PROFESSOR OF PSYCHIATRY
MEDICAL DIRECTOR, FETAL ALCOHOL EDUCATION PROGRAM
BOSTON UNIVERSITY SCHOOL OF MEDICINE

Lyn Weiner, M.P.H.
ASSOCIATE PROFESSOR OF PSYCHIATRY
(PUBLIC HEALTH)
PROGRAM DIRECTOR, FETAL ALCOHOL EDUCATION PROGRAM
BOSTON UNIVERSITY SCHOOL OF MEDICINE

New York   Oxford
OXFORD UNIVERSITY PRESS
1984

Library of Congress Cataloging in Publication Data

Rosett, Henry L.
  Alcohol and the fetus. A clinical perspective.

  Bibliography: p.
  Includes index.
  1. Fetal alcohol syndrome. 2. Fetus—Effect of drugs
on. 3. Alcohol—Physiological effect. 4. Alcoholism in
pregnancy. 5. Pregnant women—Alcohol use. I. Weiner,
Lyn. II. Title. [DNLM: 1. Alcohol drinking—In
pregnancy. 2. Alcoholic beverages—Adverse effects.
3. Fetal alcohol syndrome. 4. Fetus—Drug effects.
WQ 211 R817a]
RG629.F45R67 1984   618.3′2   84-919
ISBN 0-19-503458-9

Printed in the United States of America

Printing (last digit): 9 8 7 6 5 4 3 2

For our spouses, Atholie and Edwin,
our parents,
our children,
and the health of future generations.

Foreword

The first modern reports of the fetal alcohol syndrome (FAS) came from France in 1968. Then, in 1973, researchers at the University of Washington in Seattle independently confirmed the French observations. This stimulated a rash of case reports from around the world.

Early in 1977, while I was Director of the National Institute on Alcohol Abuse and Alcoholism (NIAAA), it became clear to us at the Institute that the time had come to collect and evaluate the growing weight of scientific evidence linking maternal drinking to impaired infants. Thus, in February of that year, we convened a workshop of eminent scientists. All the major relevant specialists were represented, including epidemiologists, biochemists, endocrinologists, pediatricians, internists, specialists in teratology, psychiatrists, and behavioral psychologists. All either were directly engaged in research on this subject or soon would be. One of the involved specialists was Dr. Henry Rosett.

The group of scientists evaluated the evidence from every vantage point possible—animal studies, case reports, metabolic and physiologic studies, epidemiology, biochemical and the behavioral sciences. After looking at all the evidence, they arrived at two interconnecting conclusions: (1) the FAS had been clinically observed in humans and (2) heavy consumption of alcohol by animals during pregnancy produced malformations in their offspring that were strikingly similar to the FAS observed in humans.

With these conclusions in hand, the scientists recommended that the NIAAA issue a Caution to the Nation that would point out the risks to unborn infants associated with drinking alcohol by the mother. This I did at a press conference held in Washington, DC, on June 1, 1977, and my statement read as follows:

> Recent research reports indicate that heavy use of alcohol by women during pregnancy may result in a pattern of abnormalities in the offspring, termed the Fetal Alcohol Syndrome, which consist of specific congenital and behavioral abnormalities. Studies undertaken in animals corroborate the initial observations in humans and indicate as well an increased incidence of stillbirths, resorptions, and spontaneous abortions. Both the risks and the extent of abnormalities appear to be dose-related, increasing with higher alcohol intake during the pregnancy period. In human studies, alcohol is an unequivocal factor when the full pattern of the FAS is present. In cases where all the characteristics are not present, the correlations between alcohol and the adverse effects are complicated by such factors as nutrition, smoking, caffeine and other drug consumption.

I concluded with this warning:

> Given the total evidence available at this time, pregnant women should be particularly conscious of the extent of their drinking. While safe levels of drinking are unknown, it appears that a risk is established with ingestion above 3 ounces of absolute alcohol or 6 drinks per day. Between 1 ounce and 3 ounces, there is still uncertainty but caution is advised. Therefore, pregnant women and those likely to become pregnant should discuss their drinking habits and the potential dangers with their physicians.

Since that Caution was released in 1977, there has been an exponential increase in animal and human studies on the FAS, not only in the U.S. but also abroad. However, little new evidence has accrued that would alter the basic message of that earlier warning. Still there are those who have taken extremist positions averring that even a sip of an alcoholic beverage would damage the unborn embryo or fetus. Others, still to this day, against overwhelming evidence, deny that FAS exists.

Henry Rosett and his colleague Lyn Weiner, modern pioneers in FAS research and education, have written an eminently readable, balanced and multidimensional book on alcohol and the fetus. They begin with a historical view of the problem and then consider the diagnostic complexities of the FAS and describe the incidence of the problem. This is followed by a discussion of drinking practices and the adult problem drinker, with special emphasis on women and the pharmacology and physiology of alcohol. The next chapter describes the maternal-placental-fetal system and the adverse effects of alcohol upon it. In Chapter 4, the authors delineate the prenatal effects of alcohol on fetal growth and describe their own prenatal study at Boston City Hospital and the positive outcome they observed when women reduced drinking during pregnancy. Chapter 5 details the effects of alcohol in producing abnormalities in organ and other systems. Moreover, it discusses important factors that influence the development of these abnormalities and their possible pathophysiologic mechanisms. The following chapter deals with alcohol's complex effects on the developing central nervous system.

Technical, methodological, and definitional issues are discussed in Chapter 7. In Chapter 8, the authors, using case reports, point to some pitfalls in intervention and therapy and suggest positive approaches to treating pregnant women who have a drinking problem. In the next chapter, using a broad clinical perspective, Rosett and Weiner point to ways of planning a pregnancy and how to avoid complications. They also suggest means for minimizing risk and consider other factors in producing a viable and healthy infant. The final chapter deals with media campaigns, professional education and what the authors consider to be realistic counselling.

The book is full of interesting and factual information, both historical and current, that should serve well the investigator, the health care professional and educator. The authors thoughtfully weave through the fabric of the book basic science, clinical and epidemiological information that relates to the FAS. It is a work that is scholarly, yet practical in scope and contains much sound advice. In an arena that is rapidly developing, where dissent, ambiguity, lack of definition and even emotionalism are prevalent, the authors do a remarkably good job of dealing with these contentious issues in an objective and reasoned manner. It is obvious to me that Henry Rosett's and Lyn Weiner's years of in-depth experience as investigators, teachers, and clinicians have been brought to full fruition in this volume. This book is a great tribute to both of its authors.

Ernest P. Noble, Ph.D., M.D.
Pike Professor of Alcohol Studies
Director, Alcohol Research Center
University of California, Los Angeles

Preface

Since the initial description of the fetal alcohol syndrome a decade ago the proliferation of knowledge about maternal alcohol consumption and fetal development has been rapid and has involved many disciplines. This stimulated us to review the international literature, integrating experimental, epidemiologic, and clinical findings with our experience at the Boston City Hospital prenatal clinic. The application of research findings to a spectrum of clinical issues is presented, with emphasis on techniques for identifying and treating women who drink heavily during pregnancy. We also consider the limitations of current knowledge and the implications for the complex decisions that must be made.

This comprehensive overview is directed primarily toward health professionals who care for pregnant women and their families. Since alcohol abuse traditionally was considered peripheral to their professional responsibilities, basic information about alcohol and fetal development is included. Effective prevention of fetal alcohol effects requires the collaboration of obstetricians, pediatricians, family practitioners, nurses, midwives, and nutritionists, who must learn to identify and counsel women at risk. Psychiatrists, psychologists, social workers, and alcoholism counselors will be called upon to help treat women who do not respond to their primary health care providers. Professionals in the educational and rehabilitation disciplines need to be aware of the special needs of FAS children and their families. This review also is directed toward individuals concerned with developing health policy and evaluating research.

The renewed interest in the adverse effects of maternal alcohol abuse on fetal development coincides with an expansion of knowledge about the biochemistry and pharmacology of alcohol. Recent research on the metabolism of alcohol and the associated pathophysiology at both cellular and neuroendocrine levels has explained the mechanisms of multiple medical problems. The fetus shares basic biochemical and structural characteristics with the adult organism, including susceptibility to adverse effects of alcohol. Disruptions of development during periods of rapid growth and organization of tissues may affect health throughout life. Research and clinical interest has expanded well beyond the pathology of the chronic alcoholic, and now considers the effects of alcohol throughout the life cycle.

Developing effective strategies to prevent the adverse effects of alcohol on mother and child requires the integration of multiple perspectives. Alcohol's biochemical and pharmacologic actions are complex but comprehensible. Psychological and sociological issues confuse clinicians and their patients as well as health planners. Confusion would be reduced by making health policy consistent with scientific facts. Therefore an objective and comprehensive synthesis is important to those seeking solutions to this significant health problem.

Our clinical, educational, and investigative activities have continued since 1974. We gratefully acknowledge financial support from many sources: a Career Teacher Award from the National Institute on Drug Abuse and Alcoholism (T01DA 00031) and the National Institute on Alcohol Abuse and Alcoholism (PHSAA 07008), Rockville, Maryland; the Charles H. Hood Foundation, the Massachusetts Public Health Trust, Trustees of Health and Hospitals of the City of Boston, and the Commonwealth of Massachusetts Developmental Disabilities Council, Boston; the National Council on Alcoholism, New York City; the United States Brewers Association, Washington, D.C.; the National Institute on Alcohol Abuse and Alcoholism (R01-AA02-446 and R01-AA0127), Rockville, Maryland; and the Licensed Beverage Information Council, Washington, D.C. Preparation of the manuscript was supported by the Distilled Spirits Council of the United States, Inc., Washington, D.C.

Many individuals contributed to the success of our program at Boston City Hospital and to this book. The staff of the Maternal Health and Child Development program at Boston City Hospital collaborated with us and provided a forum for refining ideas. Members of the Department of Obstetrics and Gynecology and of the

Division of Psychiatry of Boston City Hospital and Boston University School of Medicine have demonstrated sustained interest since the planning phase of our program. The Fetal Alcohol Study Group of the Research Society on Alcoholism freely shared ideas and experiences and broadened our understanding of many issues. This exchange of ideas encouraged collaboration among participants and contributed to progress.

We are particularly grateful to Ernest Noble, Ph.D., M.D., Carrie Randall, Ph.D., and Robert Sokol, M.D., for their critical reading of the manuscript and constructive suggestions.

Jean Kazez, our research associate, provided invaluable editorial assistance, and her literary skills contributed to the clarity of this book.

Our families' patience, encouragement, and good humor throughout the project was essential. Their sustained love and commitment has been the most important ingredient.

Boston, Massachusetts   H.L.R.
November, 1983   L.W.

Contents

ALCOHOL AND THE FETUS

One

Fetal Alcohol Syndrome

Historical background

The belief that parental consumption of alcohol at the time of conception and during pregnancy could have adverse effects on the health of offspring has a long history (Warner and Rosett, 1975). Carthage and Sparta both had laws prohibiting the use of alcohol by newly married couples to prevent them from conceiving while intoxicated. Aristotle, in his *Problemata*, wrote that "foolish, drunken, or harebrain women, for the most part bring forth children like unto themselves, *morosos et languidos*"—an observation Burton cited in *The Anatomy of Melancholy* in 1621. One hundred years later, medical concern about alcohol use during pregnancy began in England, when the traditional restrictions on distillation were lifted and the country was flooded with cheap gin. During the gin epidemic of 1720–1750, birthrates dropped and there was a sharp rise in the mortality of children under five years of age (George, 1965; Coffey, 1966). Although multiple factors must be considered, maternal drinking is a likely explanation; this was a period when crops and wages were good and epidemic disease relatively rare. In 1726 the College of Physicians petitioned Parliament to control the distilling trade, calling gin "a cause of weak, feeble and distempered children" (George, 1965).

Throughout the 19th Century, children of alcoholics were observed to have a higher frequency of mental retardation, epilepsy, stillbirths, and infant deaths. Numerous clinical and experimental research reports on the effects of alcohol on offspring appeared in both the British and American medical and biological literature. In the middle of the century, the temperance movement and medicine became closely intertwined. Medical writers were influenced by moral attitudes, and moral leaders were eager to find physiologic evidence to strengthen their arguments. Both groups stressed the idea that the sins of intemperate fathers could be visited on their children for several generations. In 1826, Lyman Beecher, a Massachusetts clergyman and an early advocate of temperance in the U.S., argued that alcohol was poisoning and debilitating the human race: "The free and universal use of intoxicating liquors for a few centuries can not fail to bring down our race from the majestic, athletic forms of our fathers, to the similitude of a despicable and puny race of men" (Beecher, 1827). Justin Edwards (1847), a friend and coworker of Beecher's, published a temperance manual stating that "the children of mothers who drink alcohol are more likely than others to become drunkards, and in various ways to suffer. Often they are not so large and healthy as other children. They have less keenness and strength of eyesight, less firmness and quietness of nerves, less capability of great bodily and mental achievement, and less power to withstand the attacks of disease, or the vicissitudes of climate and seasons."

In 1899, William Sullivan, physician to a Liverpool prison, published "A Note on the Influence of Maternal Inebriety on the Offspring," a careful study of 600 offspring of 120 alcoholic women. He located 28 nondrinking female relatives of the alcoholic women and found that the infant mortality and stillborn rate was 2½ times higher among the alcoholics' children than in the comparison population. Several alcoholic women who had had infants with severe and often fatal complications later bore healthy children when imprisonment forced them to abstain from alcohol during pregnancy.

By the turn of the century a vast body of epidemiologic research had accumulated on the relationship between parental drinking and "mental degeneracy" in children. Once the 18th amendment was ratified and Prohibition went into effect in 1920, however, medical concern about alcohol and pregnancy dropped dramatically. Medical researchers, like many Americans, believed that alcohol was now a dead issue. With the exception of a few animal experiments, studies on alcohol's effects on offspring virtually disappeared until 1940. When interest in the topic revived, scientists discounted and ridiculed the pre-Prohibition literature, charging that the early epidemiologic research had had "an axe to grind" and that the animal experiments had been crude and uncontrolled. Because of its moralistic and unscientific language, researchers tended to overlook valuable ideas in the medical temperance literature.

In 1942, Haggard and Jellinek stated that damage occurred in the reproductive organs of chronic alcoholics, but that there was no evidence of damage to human germ cells. The possibility of intra-uterine effects of alcohol was not considered. Poor nutrition in the alcoholic mother and the disturbance of home life created by parental alcoholism were blamed for abnormalities observed among children. For the next several decades most researchers dismissed the idea that alcohol had prenatal effects, and they accepted environmental explanations for abnormalities found in children of heavy drinkers.

While American research was in a lull, French and German researchers in the 50s and 60s continued to report higher frequencies of neurologic disorders, together with delays in growth and development, in the offspring of alcoholic parents (Heuyer et al, 1957; Christiaens et al, 1960). Lemoine et al (1968) studied 127 children from 69 French families in which there was chronic alcoholism. In 29 families both parents were alcoholics, in 25 only the mother was, and in 15 only the father. Twenty-five children had malformations: five, cleft palates; three, micro-ophthalmia; six, limb malformations; seven, congenital heart disease; and four, visceral anomalies. They shared common facial profiles, including protruding foreheads, sunken nasal bridges, short, upturned noses, retracted upper lips, receding chins, and deformed ears. Many were hyperactive, with delayed psychomotor and language development. As these children grew older, they had difficulty sustaining an activity for a period of time and had behavior problems in school. Their average IQ was 70. Lemoine et al attributed the adverse outcomes to the in utero exposure to alcohol which resulted from maternal alcoholism. Their article was neglected by American researchers and clinicians even though an abstract was published in English (National Foundation, 1968).

In the United States, awareness of alcohol-related birth defects was stimulated by a report in 1970 that 10 out of 12 offspring of 11 alcoholic women were small for gestational age and failed to grow even with adequate diets (Ulleland et al, 1970). Five of the 10 were developmentally retarded as tested by the Gessell or Denver developmental scales. Jones et al (1973) recognized a specific pattern of malformations in four of these children and in an additional seven offspring of alcoholic mothers. They coined the term "fetal alcohol syndrome" (FAS) to describe the pattern of prenatal and postnatal growth deficiency, developmental delay or mental deficiency, microcephaly, and fine motor dysfunction. The children had characteristic facies with short palpebral fissures, micro-ophthalmia, midfacial hypoplasia, and epicanthal folds. A significant number had abnormal palmar creases, minor joint anomalies, cardiac defects, anomalies of the external genitalia, small hemangiomas, and minor ear anomalies.

Diagnosis of FAS

The initial publications that identified and described the fetal alcohol syndrome stimulated case reports from around the world. Findings from 65 patients evaluated in Seattle and 180 cases reported from other centers helped establish minimal criteria for the diagnosis of FAS (Clarren and Smith, 1978). The routine use of these criteria was recommended by the Fetal Alcohol Study Group of the Research Society on Alcoholism (Rosett, 1980a): "The diagnosis of FAS should be made only when the patient has signs in each of these three categories:

1. Prenatal and/or postnatal growth retardation (weight, length, and/or head circumference below the tenth percentile when corrected for gestational age).

2. Central nervous system involvement (signs of neurological abnormality, developmental delay, or intellectual impairment).

3. Characteristic facial dysmorphology with at least two of these three signs: (a) microcephaly (head circumference below the third percentile), (b) micro-opthalmia and/or short palpebral fissures, (c) poorly developed philtrum, thin upper lip, and/or flattening of the maxillary area."

Retarded growth in weight, length, and head circumference both before and after birth is the most common sign of FAS. While some studies have associated prematurity with maternal alcohol use, the observed growth retardation is not merely a reflection of prematurity. FAS infants are significantly smaller than nonaffected infants after adjustment for gestational age. Postnatally, growth retardation persists even though nutrition is adequate and the environment is stable. In contrast, most children who fail to thrive for nutritional or environmental reasons respond with a growth spurt when provided with adequate nutrition in a stable environment. Catch-up growth has been demonstrated only in children with milder forms of FAS (see Chapter 4).

Mental retardation, attention deficits, delays in motor development, hyperactivity, and sleep disturbances have been observed in patients with FAS. The severity of a child's mental disorder appears to correspond to the severity of the facial dysmorphology (Streissguth et al, 1978a; Dupuis et al, 1978; Majewski, 1981). This has important prognostic implications: children with severe facial dysmorphology often show little improvement over time, whereas those with milder facial anomalies respond more favorably to therapeutic intervention and training programs. The effects of in utero exposure to alcohol on the developing central nervous system (CNS) and the underlying mechanisms are discussed in detail in Chapter 6.

The distinctive facial dysmorphology of children with FAS most often involves the eyes, nose, lip, and mid-face, but can also affect the forehead, chin, and ears (Fig. 1-1). The eyes are small, with short palpebral fissures (eye openings), epicanthal folds, ptosis (drooping eye lids) and strabismus (crossed eyes). The nose is often short and upturned with a low nasal bridge. The maxillary area is flat. The upper lip is thin, the Cupid's Bow is absent. The philtrum, two ridges between the nasal septum and upper lip, is

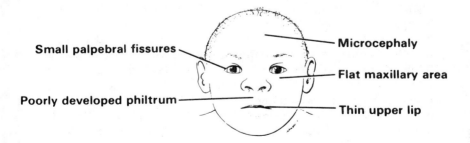

Fig. 1-1. Characteristic facial dysmorphology. (Reprinted with permission from the American College of Obstetricians and Gynecologists, *Obstet Gynecol* 57(1):1–7, 1981.)

poorly developed. The area between the nose and upper lip appears elongated. In some cases, the forehead seems to bulge and the mandible is underdeveloped. Occasionally the ears are low-set with posterior rotation.

The discipline of dysmorphology helped to define specific facial characteristics which had been vaguely described as unusual facies by other clinicians. Dysmorphologists demonstrated the importance of carefully observing subtle differences in the mid-face and eyes. Most of these characteristics represent growth failure in the mid-face which may reflect abnormal brain growth (Frias et al, 1982). Microcephaly, a failure of skull growth, also indicates small brain size. Experimental evidence is discussed in Chapter 6.

Majewski (1979), describing abnormalities similar to those observed in FAS cases, introduced the term "alcohol embryopathy" (AE), hypothesizing that the anomalies are associated with alcohol exposure during the embryonic stage of development. He devised a scoring system to differentiate mild (AEI), moderate (AEII), and severe (AEIII) cases by rating 26 anomalies associated with in utero alcohol exposure (Table 1-1). This system of classification is helpful; however, the term "FAS" seems preferable to "AE" since there is evidence that high doses of alcohol cause damage throughout gestation.

While FAS is a clinically recognizable syndrome, the diagnosis is not based on a single distinctive feature or biochemical, chromosomal, or pathological test, and it may not always be determined in the neonate. Neurological impairment may not be noticed until the child's cognitive skills are tested. Growth retardation may become obvious when the child fails to thrive despite adequate nutrition in a supportive environment. Facial dysmorphology may be difficult to recognize in the neonate. Although some have stated that dysmorphic features in the newborn are sufficiently distinct to facilitate immediate identification of FAS (Clarren, 1981), diagnosis is difficult when cases of FAS are mild and when the investigator is not experienced in distinguishing subtle differences in facies of newborns. At Boston City Hospital, four of five diagnosed cases were not identified at birth, but were subsequently recognized during routine followup care (Rosett et al, 1983b).

The combination of facial dysmorphology, growth retardation, and CNS involvement is not unique to FAS. A comparable syndrome (fetal hydantoin) is seen in the offspring of epileptic women who

Table 1-1   Symptoms in alcohol embryopathy

POINTS	SYMPTOMS
4	Intrauterine growth retardation
4	Microcephaly
2/4/8	Mental retardation
4	Hyperactivity
2	Muscular hypotonia
2	Epicanthic folds
2	Ptosis
2	Blepharophimosis
—	Antimongoloid fissures
3	Short upturned nose
1	Nasolabial furrows
1	Small lips
2	Hypoplasia of mandible
2	High arched palate
4	Cleft palate
3	Anomalous palmar creases
2	Clinodactyly, fifth finger
2	Camptodactyly
1	Hypoplasia of terminal phalanges
2	Limited supination of elbow
2	Hip dislocation
—	Pectus excavatum
4	Heart defect
2/4	Genital anomalies
1	Sacral dimple
—	Hemangiomas
2	Hernias
4	Urinary tract malformations

AEI: 10–29 points
AEII: 30–39 points
AEIII: 40 points and above

Adapted from Majewski, 1981.

have taken anticonvulsant drugs (Hill, 1976). Similar characteristics are also found in children of women with phenylketonuria (Pratt, 1980). Patients with Cornelia DeLange syndrome show uniquely shaped lips and mouth, hirsutism, short stature, and mental retardation. Noonan's syndrome involves facial features of ptosis, flat nose, and antimongoloid slant, as well as short stature, webbing of the neck, and congenital heart disease (Spiegel et al, 1979). Differentiating FAS from these syndromes is difficult without a diagnosis of maternal alcoholism. Although it is inappropriate to define cause and effect simultaneously in research programs, in clinical situations etiology can only be established with a careful history of maternal alcohol consumption and other risk factors.

Many diverse variables can inhibit the growth of the developing fetus and cause congenital abnormalities. These risk factors include maternal illness, poor nutrition, cigarette, opiate, and other drug use as well as genetic mutations, chromosomal aberrations, radiation and other environmental agents. These causal factors can act singly or synergistically. Since there are a limited number of patterns of tissue response, abnormalities which result from exposure to one or more of these variables may be similar. Specificity of abnormalities is related to the developmental stage at the time of exposure as well as to the properties of the teratogen.

Incidence of FAS

More than 400 cases of FAS have been reported in the scientific literature from all over the world, including Australia, Belgium, Brazil, Canada, Chile, Czechoslovakia, England, France, Germany, Hungary, Ireland, Italy, Japan, South Africa, Spain, Sweden, Switzerland, the U.S.S.R., and the U.S. (Abel, 1982b). The mothers represent almost every ethnic group and a broad spectrum of socioeconomic backgrounds and dietary patterns. All reported cases of the full FAS have occurred in children of chronic alcoholic mothers who drank heavily throughout pregnancy; none have been reported in children of women who drank moderately. Majewski (1981) observed that the severity depended on the stage of maternal alcoholism and not on the absolute amount of alcohol consumed. The more severely affected children (AEII or AEIII) were born to women in the later stages of alcoholism (the crucial or chronic stages as defined by Jellinek, 1960). The few offspring of women in the early phase who were affected were all diagnosed as AEI.

Not all children of mothers drinking in the alcoholic range demonstrate FAS; case reports suggest incidence rates of 33% (Dehaene et al, 1977b) and 40% (Jones et al, 1974; Majewski, 1981). Rates derived from prospective studies are markedly lower. In a cohort of 12,127 women in Cleveland, Sokol et al (1981) identified five FAS children among the offspring of 204 heavy drinkers—an incidence rate of 2.5%. In our study at Boston City Hospital there were five known cases of FAS among the offspring of 52 women who drank heavily throughout pregnancy—an incidence rate of 10% (Rosett et al, 1983b). Incidence reports in the total population are even more difficult to specify because of variabilities in study populations and differences in research methodology. Several investigators have estimated that there are 1–3 cases per 1000 live births (Dehaene et al, 1977a; Hanson et al, 1978; Dupuis et al, 1978; Olegård et al, 1979). A higher frequency has been suggested for American Indians living on reservations (Aase, 1981; May and Hymbaugh, 1982). In Cleveland, the five FAS cases observed among 12,127 newborns represent an incidence rate of about 1/2500. Based on a conservative incidence rate of one case of FAS per 1500–2000 live births, Brandt (1982) has estimated that there will be 1800–2400 new cases each year in the United States.

Clinical observations and prospective studies suggest a wide range of alcohol's effects on the developing embryo and fetus, with FAS at the far end of the spectrum. FAS cases have a higher frequency of nonspecific malformations than the general population. Associated abnormalities have been observed in ocular, oral, skeletal, cutaneous, cardiac, renal, hepatic, and immune systems, but their frequency is unclear (see Chapter 5). When frequencies are estimated from several series of case reports, one must recognize that different clinicians may use different criteria for measuring malformations and determining what is abnormal. Since published case histories usually report on the most severe or unusual form of FAS, it is possible that problems unrelated to alcohol use may be falsely associated with it. Data on nonspecific malformations must be evaluated critically; precise incidence rates are difficult to determine.

Fetal alcohol effects

Some children of alcoholics do not show the full FAS but exhibit components of the syndrome. When this has occurred in the absence of signs in all three of the areas required to diagnose FAS, the term "possible fetal alcohol effects" (FAE) has been applied. Some prefer the label "alcohol-related birth defects" when there is evidence of heavy maternal drinking and the pattern of abnormalities resembles FAS. The anomaly most commonly observed has been growth retardation. Because other risk factors have been associated with many of these effects, care must be taken to differentiate the effects of alcohol from the effects of malnutrition, other drugs, cigarettes, and genetics. It is important that parents of abnormal children not be burdened with unnecessary guilt for having consumed small amounts of alcohol and not hold themselves responsible for causing anomalies that were actually due to other causes.

Incidence rates of FAE (or alcohol-related birth defects) are difficult to determine since adverse effects often can not be directly attributed to alcohol. However, it is likely that FAE occurs far more frequently than FAS and thus represents a more widespread health problem. Brandt (1982) has estimated the incidence of FAE at 36,000 cases per year in the United States. Sokol (1981) suggests that prenatal alcohol exposure is associated with approximately 5% of all congenital anomalies.

The occurrence of abnormalities associated with FAS represents a continuum which should be studied through an epidemiological model that recognizes the role of other risk factors.

Summary

During the years following the identification and description of the fetal alcohol syndrome, there has been growing recognition of the adverse effects on offspring of heavy drinking during pregnancy. Within a relatively brief period, a body of new research findings has developed that is consistent with research and clinical observations dating back to the 18th Century. The scientific attitude toward these data has shifted from skepticism to recognition of a major health problem. In our society people have intense feelings about alcohol abuse, maternal responsibility, and child welfare. Consequently there has been a tendency for research findings to be seized upon, interpreted, and used by well-intentioned groups with a variety of social goals. By carefully examining the data first, the historical cycle of acceptance and rejection of findings about alcohol's effects on fetal development can be avoided. Only with scientific objectivity can we untangle the interacting metabolic, environmental, and social variables.

Two

Alcohol and the Adult

The discovery of beverage alcohol probably occurred soon after waterproof pots were developed and used to store and transport water and fruit. Spontaneous fermentation of grains, fruits, and sugars produced liquids which were found to enhance pleasure. During the Middle Ages, alchemists discovered that distillation increased this power and thought they had found the elixir of life. Alcoholic beverages have been produced and consumed by almost every culture since prehistoric times and their use and abuse have been recorded for millennia.

Most cultures have sanctions for the use of alcohol within their religious and social structure, with limits imposed on the amount consumed and the permissible degree of intoxication. Society's restrictions on the availability of alcohol range from heavy taxes and limited distribution to prohibition. Generally, there is disapproval of levels of drinking that lead to violent behavior or loss of self-control, and of drinking that contributes to absenteeism, high accident rates, or poor work performance.

In the United States, 75% of males and 60% of females report drinking at least occasionally (USDHHS, 1981). Approximately 90% of those who consume alcohol do not have a problem regulating its use.

Patterns of pathologic alcohol use have been classified as alcohol abuse and alcohol dependence in the American Psychiatric Association's Diagnostic and Statistical Manual of Mental Disorders (DSMIII).

Patterns of pathologic use include: need for daily use of alcohol for adequate functioning; inability to cut down or stop drinking; repeated efforts to control or reduce excess drinking by periods of temporary abstinence or restricting drinking to certain times of the day; binges (remaining intoxicated throughout the day for at least two days); occasional consumption of a fifth of spirits or its equivalent in wine or beer; amnesic periods for events occurring while intoxicated (blackouts); continuation of drinking despite a serious physical disorder that the individual knows is exacerbated by alcohol use; drinking of non-beverage alcohol. These patterns of pathological use result in impairment of social and occupational functioning. When this pattern persists for at least one month, the criteria for alcohol abuse are met. Alcohol dependence is diagnosed when signs of tolerance or withdrawal occur. Tolerance is marked by the need for increased amounts of alcohol to achieve the desired effect. Early signs of withdrawal include shakes and malaise relieved by drinking. More advanced withdrawal includes coarse tremor, rapid heart beat, elevated blood pressure, and sweating.

"Alcohol dependence" in DSMIII was considered preferable to the term "alcoholism," which often is used without standardized criteria and elicits pessimistic and moralistic reactions. However, some want to retain the term "alcoholism" since it is widely accepted and understood and is essential for legislation that has established treatment and rehabilitation programs.

The incidence of alcohol abuse varies with demographic characteristics, including age, sex, ethnicity, and geographic area. Alcohol dependence is most prevalent among men aged 21–34. Women in the reproductive years (ages 21–49) drink more heavily than older women (USDHHS, 1981).

Alcohol and women

Differences in alcohol use between men and women, once dramatic, are narrowing and disappearing. Historically, social controls on alcohol consumption have been stricter for women than for men. Drinking, especially problem drinking, contradicts social ideals of feminine behavior. As mothers, women are expected to be responsible, nurturing, and selfless. When the alcohol-dependent woman is judged by these standards, she meets with disapproval instead of compassion. New roles for women have changed some of society's expectations; nonetheless moral condemnation of female alcohol abusers remains common among laymen and professionals.

DRINKING PATTERNS AMONG PREGNANT WOMEN

In our study at Boston City Hospital of alcohol consumption by pregnant women, we classified women as rare, moderate, or heavy drinkers (Rosett et al, 1978). We adapted the method of Cahalan et al (1969) who surveyed American drinking practices and standardized a Quantity-Frequency-Variability Index which assesses the average volume consumed daily and whether drinking is "massed" or "spaced." Heavy drinkers in our study satisfied criteria for "high-volume, high-maximum" drinking: consumption of at least five drinks on some occasions and a minimum daily average of 1½ drinks. Moderate drinkers included all women who drank more than once a month but did not meet the criteria for heavy drinking. Rare drinkers used alcohol less than once a month and never consumed five drinks on any occasion. These definitions only mark off boundaries in a spectrum of drinking patterns. Among 1711 women, 53% drank rarely or not at all, 37% drank moderately, and 9% were heavy drinkers (Weiner et al, 1983).

Many definitions of drinking patterns have been used in studies of alcohol consumption reported by pregnant women. In Cleveland, women were differentiated on the basis of their responses to the Michigan Alcoholism Screening Test (MAST) (Selzer, 1971; Sokol et al, 1981). Researchers at Loma Linda defined heavy drinking as an average daily consumption of at least 2 oz absolute alcohol (AA) (Kuzma and Kissinger, 1981). In France, heavy drinkers were defined as women who reported drinking more than 400 ml of wine (1.5 oz AA) per day (Kaminski et al, 1976). In Ottawa, a woman was considered to be a heavy social drinker if she reported a daily average greater than 0.85 oz AA (Fried et al, 1980). In Seattle, heavy drinkers were women who reported a daily average of more than 1.0 oz AA (Streissguth et al, 1981). A study in northern California defined heavy drinking as a daily minimum average of 1–2 drinks (0.5–1.0 oz AA) (Harlap and Shiono, 1980). In Sweden, women who reported consuming between 1 and 8.3 oz (30–125 g) a day were considered excessive drinkers and women reporting over 8.3 oz were classified as alcohol abusers (Larsson, 1983). Despite the different definitions, each project identified a group of women, ranging from 2–14% of the sample, who reported drinking significantly more than the rest of the study population (Weiner et al, 1983). This is consistent with the results of a survey representative of the whole population in which 5–7% of pregnant women reported getting drunk or drinking five or more drinks on some occasions (Opinion Research Corporation, 1979).

Drinking patterns are commonly described in a linear fashion although the distribution of quantity consumed is rarely linear. At Boston City Hospital, moderate drinkers reported consuming a daily average of 0.3 oz AA (range 0.01–3.6 oz). Heavy drinkers reported a mean daily consumption of 4.6 oz AA (range 0.8–27.0 oz), an amount 15 times greater than the moderate. Distribution of consumption within the groups was skewed, with 27% of the heavy drinkers reporting daily averages above the mean. Thus, the mean score reflects high levels of consumption for a relatively small portion (27%) of the heavy drinkers. Disproportionately high mean daily scores have been reported by the heaviest drinkers in Cleveland (2.0 oz AA) and Loma Linda (5.9 oz AA). Means were not included in reports from other programs.

Variability in drinking was reported by the women at Boston City Hospital. At the time of registration for care, 37% of the women reported changes in their drinking habits throughout life and in the early stages of pregnancy. Three percent reported that their current levels of drinking were higher than at any other time in their lives; 34% reported that their current consumption was lower. The women reporting lower levels of alcohol use represent 30% of the abstinent or rare group, 35% of the moderate, and 60% of the heavy drinking group. Similar changes in alcohol consumption throughout pregnancy with marked reductions among heavy drinkers have been noted by others. Reduction in alcohol use from pre-pregnancy levels was reported by 50% of the women interviewed in Seattle (Little et al, 1976; Little and Streissguth, 1978). The women defined as heavy drinkers decreased their consumption more than the others but remained the heaviest drinkers in the sample. In Cleveland, reduction in consumption was reported by 50% of the women who met criteria for alcohol abuse (Sokol et al, 1981). The Ottawa study reported that 37% of the women changed their self-report of alcohol use sufficiently to move to lower drinking categories between pre-pregnancy and pregnancy (Fried et al, 1980). Among heavy social drinkers, 66% reduced alcohol consumption. In the Swedish study, alcohol intake was reduced by all the "excessive" drinkers and 78% of the alcohol abusers (Larsson, 1983). In the Loma Linda study, 11.4% of the women reported that they stopped drinking for one or two trimesters (Kuzma and Kissinger, 1981). Reduction of alcohol use by the heavy drinkers was not described separately. A study of abortions in a poor, urban population revealed that 38% of the cases and 65% of the controls decreased drinking from pre-pregnancy levels (Kline et al, 1980). In a Los Angeles County survey of a sample representative of the broad spectrum of women giving birth, 58% reported decreased drinking during pregnancy (Minor and Van Dort, 1982).

Among the 162 women classified as heavy drinkers at Boston City Hospital, the frequency and quantity of drinking varied. Daily drinking was reported by 64%; 21% drank 3–4 times a week, and 10% drank 1–2 times a week. Few reported consuming the same amount each day. Most had a beverage of choice: 39% preferred beer, 30% drank liquor, 16% combined beer and liquor. Few drank wine.

PROBLEM DRINKERS

The stereotype of the typical female problem drinker is the older housewife, who drinks alone at home, her consumption "hidden" from the outside world. In fact, women's heavy drinking is not more hidden than men's. It occurs most often among younger, single, divorced, and separated women regardless of employment status (Mello, 1980). Most relevant to alcohol and the fetus are the differences between women who drink heavily during childbearing years and those who do not. A review of prospective studies of drinking patterns among pregnant women demonstrated that those who drank heavily shared a cluster of behavioral characteristics (Weiner et al, 1983). Heavy drinking was consistently associated with increased age, parity, cigarette smoking, and use of other drugs, such as marijuana, heroin, barbiturates, psychedelics, and amphetamines. In addition, heavy-drinking women were exposed to more social stress. They were less apt to be married and more apt to associate with others who drank heavily.

Antecedents of alcohol dependence are nonspecific: no single factor has been identified that can predict alcohol abuse or explain why some people develop drinking problems and others do not. People drink heavily for a variety of reasons, and problems with alcohol can develop in anyone who uses large amounts of alcohol over a long period of time. At one time, female alcoholics were thought to be more psychologically disturbed and more socially deviant than males. Current research, however, points to the fact that although depression is seen more commonly in alcohol-dependent females than in males, abusers of both sexes exhibit a range of pre-alcoholic personalities (Mello, 1980). As drinking progresses, the so called "alcoholic personality" develops as a result of alcohol's effects on memory and judgment and the influence of living in a subculture in which drinking is a central activity.

Interactions between endocrine, physiologic, behavioral, and affective factors may influence the development of problem drinking by women. Variations in blood alcohol concentrations during different phases of the menstrual cycle may affect drinking patterns and their reinforcement (Mello, 1980). During pregnancy, maternal changes may modify the metabolism of, and the physiologic response to, alcohol. These interactions have not been studied intensively and need more exploration.

The frequency of alcohol problems is higher in families of alcoholics than in families of nonalcoholics. Genetics have been implicated in studies of males; however, environmental factors seem to have a greater influence on females. Although the etiologic roles of genetic and environmental factors have been assessed, little consideration has been given to the additional effects of in utero alcohol exposure.

The Copenhagen Adoption Study of alcoholism among 55 adopted sons and 49 adopted daughters of alcoholic natural parents found that alcoholism increased in sons but not in daughters as compared with adopted offspring of nonalcoholics (Goodwin, 1971; Goodwin et al, 1973). Cases were included if one parent had a hospital diagnosis of alcoholism; in 85% it was the father. Information on the drinking patterns of the other parent was not reported. Since couples often share drinking behaviors, many wives probably were drinking heavily also, even though they had not been hospitalized or diagnosed as alcoholic. Thus, late behavioral manifestations of the effects of alcohol in utero may have been attributed to genetic influences. A study of 913 Swedish women adopted by non-relatives at an early age (Bohman et al, 1981) supports this possibility. A three-fold excess of alcohol abusers was found among women with alcoholic biological mothers as compared with daughters of nonalcoholic parents. When separate effects of maternal and paternal alcoholism were examined, the maternal influence accounted for twice as much of the variance as the paternal influence. The researchers suggest that the alcoholic mother exerts a greater influence because she provides the intrauterine environment as well as genetic background.

Pharmacology of alcohol

Beverage alcohol (ethyl alcohol or ethanol) is a simple molecule, C_2H_5OH, with a molecular weight of 46. It is soluble in water and lipids and rapidly distributes throughout the total body water, quickly crossing both the blood–brain barrier and the placental barrier. Ethyl alcohol contains two carbon atoms. Other alcohols with carbon chains of various lengths (e.g., one carbon=methyl, three carbons=propyl) are present in small amounts in some alcoholic beverages. In this book, as in common usage, the term "alcohol" refers to ethyl alcohol.

When yeast grows without air in carbohydrate solution, sugars are fermented to alcohol and carbon dioxide. When the alcohol concentration approximates 12%, the alcohol itself inhibits growth of the yeast and the process stops. Fortified wines such as sherry, port, and muscatel are produced by adding alcohol to raise the concentration to about 20%. Beer, produced by fermenting grain and hops, is usually 3–5% alcohol. Various types of liquor are produced by fermenting grain, corn, potatoes, or sugar cane. Distillation raises the concentration of alcohol, usually to 40% or 50%, although it can be increased to 95%. Alcohol content is described in the U.S. as "proof," which is double the alcohol concentration. Thus an 80 proof vodka is 40% alcohol.

Although beer, wine, and liquor vary in alcohol concentration, the alcohol content of a drink of each beverage can be standardized to 0.5 oz (15 ml) of absolute alcohol (AA). Since the concentration of alcohol in beer is approximately 4%, the usual 12 oz can contains about 0.5 oz AA. The concentration of alcohol in table wine is approximately 12%: a 4 oz glass contains 0.5 oz AA. One hundred proof

whiskey is 50% alcohol: 1 oz contains 0.5 oz AA. The volume of
beverages of various concentrations that contains a standard drink
can be computed easily: for example 0.5 oz AA is contained in 1.2 oz
of an 80 proof beverage or in 2.5 oz of fortified wine (40 proof).

By evaluating alcohol consumption in terms of these standard
drinks, clinicians can quickly estimate the total amount of alcohol
ingested. However, people do not measure their alcohol with the
precision used in the laboratory: self-reports should always be recognized as approximations. When reports of alcohol consumption
are quantified to several decimal points, scientists create an illusion
of unattainable precision.

BLOOD ALCOHOL CONCENTRATION

A clinical understanding of the pharmacology of ethanol is facilitated by approximations which, like estimates of consumption, are
imprecise. Ethanol has a specific gravity close to that of water; thus
every milliliter weighs about 1 gram. A drink (0.5 oz AA) contains
about 15 grams of ethanol. Upon consumption it is rapidly distributed
throughout the total body water (about 60% of the body weight). A
130 pound person (59 kg) contains about 35 liters of water. Fifteen
grams of ethanol in 35 liters of water equals 43 grams per 100 liters.
This blood alcohol concentration (BAC) may be expressed as 43
mg/100 ml, or 43 mg percent, or 0.043 g/100 ml which is by conven-
tion rounded to 0.04. In most states, a BAC of 0.10 is legally defined as
the lower limit of intoxication. A 130 pound woman will have a BAC
of 0.10 after consuming three drinks within one hour.

In nonaddicted drinkers, blood alcohol levels can be roughly
correlated to mental state with variability between individuals. Mild
euphoria exists at 30 mg percent; impaired coordination may become manifest with 50 mg percent; and ataxia is often apparent at
100 mg percent. Stupors can occur at 300 mg percent and narcosis
and death at 400 mg percent. Alcoholics and heavy drinkers who
have developed physiologic tolerance are often able to coordinate
walking and to seem alert at 300 mg percent, even though their
judgment and complex responses are severely impaired.

Slightly higher peak BACs are found in women than in men
consuming the same quantity of alcohol. Females have more fatty
tissue and less lean muscle mass than males; since there is less water

in fatty tissue than in muscle, the alcohol is diluted in a smaller volume. Differences in the volume of body water as well as in estrogen and progesterone levels at various stages of the menstrual cycle also cause small changes in the BAC in response to an equivalent dose (Jones and Jones, 1976). Similarly, changes in body water and hormone levels during pregnancy may affect the BAC. These physiologic differences cause a relatively small variability in BACs, however, compared to the great variability resulting from differences in the quantity consumed.

METABOLISM OF ALCOHOL

Following ingestion, some 20–30% of the alcohol is rapidly absorbed through the stomach wall. The balance mixes with gastric acids and mucous and is absorbed through the small intestine. It diffuses from the stomach and intestine to the blood vessels and is carried by the portal vein to the liver. Once alcohol is distributed throughout the body water, more than 95% is oxidized, while small amounts are excreted unchanged in the breath, urine, and sweat. The liver is the main site of ethanol oxidation, although the kidney, muscle, lung, and intestine metabolize small quantities.

Oxidation of ethyl alcohol occurs in several stages. The first step is the oxidation of ethanol to acetaldehyde, which is catalyzed mainly by the enzyme alcohol dehydrogenase. (Additional enzyme systems may account for 10–20% of ethanol oxidation.) In the second step, catalyzed by the enzyme aldehyde dehydrogenase, acetaldehyde is oxidized to acetate. Each of these oxidative steps is coupled with the reduction of the coenzyme nicotinamide adenine dinucleotide (NAD) to NADH. Acetate is then oxidized to water and carbon dioxide through the Krebs cycle of intermediate metabolism.

The rate of metabolism of ethanol is governed by zero order kinetics. The BAC falls at approximately 15 mg percent per hour, regardless of the initial BAC. The rate-limiting step is the oxidation of ethanol to acetaldehyde. After one standard drink, the 130 pound person has an initial BAC of about 43 mg percent, which will fall to approximately 28 mg percent in an hour and will be close to zero in three hours. These approximations assume that all of the alcohol is consumed at once and is absorbed quickly. The presence of food in the stomach and the speed at which the beverage is consumed affect the rate of increase of the BAC but not the rate of metabolism. Similarly, although the same quantity of alcohol will cause slightly higher BACs in women than in men of equal weight, no sexual differences have been observed in the rate of metabolism.

The human liver (and that of other mammals) is rich in alcohol dehydrogenase. It functions to oxidize the ethanol that is spontaneously produced within the intestine by microorganisms that ferment carbohydrates (Blomstrand, 1971). Lester (1961, 1962), on the basis of his own research and a review of other experiments, concluded that humans and most mammals endogenously produce about 12–39 g of alcohol in 24 hours. In abstinent men, the endogenously produced blood ethanol concentration in the portal vein was measured at 0.08 mg percent (Sprung et al, 1981). This level of alcohol is probably oxidized during its first pass through the hepatic circulation. Very small amounts of alcohol—such as those ingested in a dose of cough medicine—are probably also oxidized rapidly by the hepatic alcohol dehydrogenase.

Aldehyde dehydrogenase functions primarily in the liver, although small amounts are present in virtually every organ in the body. The hepatic capacity to oxidize acetaldehyde is extremely efficient; no concentrations can be measured in the circulation following light or moderate alcohol consumption. With elevated BACs, high concentrations occur. These levels remain steady over a wide range of falling ethanol levels but drop sharply when the concentration of ethanol reaches about 24 μM (110 mg percent) (Korsten et al, 1975). Acetaldehyde levels greater than 35 μM per liter are responsible for some of the pathologic damage associated with alcoholism. The toxicity of acetaldehyde results from its high level of reactivity with other organic molecules and its lipid solubility. In rat liver microsomes, binding of acetaldehyde to proteins is enhanced after chronic alcohol consumption (Nomura and Lieber, 1981).

Alcoholics demonstrate higher levels of acetaldehyde than nonalcoholics drinking equivalent amounts (Korsten et al, 1975). When alcohol abuse stops and nutrition is adequate, the disproportionately high blood acetaldehyde levels no longer occur (Lindros, 1975). High acetaldehyde levels secondary to chronic alcohol ingestion reflect a capacity for increased production, accomplished by additional ethanol-oxidizing enzymes, as well as impaired liver aldehyde dehydrogenase activity.

Individuals also vary in their capacity to metabolize acetaldehyde because of genetic differences in enzyme systems (Von Wartburg, 1980; Lindros, 1983). People with "atypical" alcohol dehydrogenase have elevated acetaldehyde levels, accompanied by flushing of the skin. Although this has been reported most commonly among Orientals, it also occurs frequently in American Indians. It has also been observed in individuals who lack one of the aldehyde dehydrogenase isoenzymes (Agarawal et al, 1981). Genetic aldehyde dehydrogenase deficiency impairs the ability to remove acetaldehyde and may contribute to alcohol intolerance.

The acquired ability to consume large quantities of alcohol, so striking among alcoholics, develops from CNS tolerance to higher BACs as well as induction of additional oxidizing capacity (Von Wartburg, 1971; Lieber and DiCarli, 1972). Within the liver, induction of the microsomal ethanol oxidizing system (MEOS) supplements alcohol dehydrogenase. MEOS oxidative capacity, relatively small among moderate drinkers, increases as alcoholism develops and can contribute as much as 50% of metabolism in heavy drinkers. Since the MEOS also oxidizes other sedative drugs, a cross-tolerance to various sedatives develops.

Tolerance is associated with physiologic alterations of the CNS which facilitate relatively normal functioning despite high alcohol concentrations. One mechanism of tolerance involves nonspecific changes in the fluidity of cell membranes through alteration in the structure of the lipo-protein bilayer. This can alter membrane potentials and excitability. Multiple metabolic changes within the CNS may cause withdrawal reactions when the BAC falls. Mild withdrawal, experienced as the irritability of a hangover, is typically relieved by a few more drinks the morning after. Withdrawal reactions following long periods of heavy drinking can be much more severe and include tremulousness, convulsions, and delerium tremens (DTs). Gastrointestinal disturbances and irritability often occur. These symptoms usually subside within a few days, but can persist for a week or more. Sleep disturbances have been observed in chronic alcoholics as long as 200 weeks after abstinence was achieved (Wagman and Allen, 1975). The cycle of tolerance and withdrawal creates an addictive mechanism: the person who initially drank to modify moods and thoughts requires increasing quantities to relieve the unpleasant symptoms caused by the alcohol itself and its withdrawal.

Alcohol's physiologic effects

The consumption of small amounts of alcohol (in the range of two drinks) causes no permanent physiologic alterations. Alcohol in higher concentrations modifies cell functions throughout the body, affecting all organ systems. Following acute ingestion, the physiologic changes are reversible, but with chronic abuse they may result in permanent damage. Oxidation of large amounts of alcohol results in the release of excess hydrogen ions which alter the NAD/ NADH ratio and change the oxidation-reduction potential of liver cells. Multiple alterations in the intermediate metabolism of carbohydrates, proteins, and fats result. For example, the process whereby amino acids are converted into glucose, with pyruvate as an intermediate, is turned in a different direction. Instead of being converted into glucose, the pyruvate is reduced to lactate. There also is an increased breakdown of glycogen stored in the tissues and an impairment in the formation of new glycogen. When an alcoholic person no longer synthesizes glucose from amino acids, and glycogen stores in the liver become exhausted, hypoglycemia or low blood sugar results. Lactate builds up, producing lactic acidosis. Changes in the formation of lipids result in deposition of large quantities of fat in the liver. Some excess fats are converted into ketone bodies, and the resulting ketoacidosis resembles that of uncontrolled diabetes. During pregnancy, these alterations can adversely affect the environment in which the fetus develops.

GASTROINTESTINAL SYSTEM

Alcohol is both a drug and a food. Its metabolism produces 7 calories per gram or approximately 105 calories per standard drink. When a pregnant woman consumes 10 drinks a day, the alcohol itself provides almost half of her required daily calories. However, alcohol provides few, if any, vitamins, minerals, or proteins. Other components of alcoholic beverages contribute varying amounts of additional calories and nutrients. Beer contains significant amounts of at least 10 amino acids, as well as nicotinamide. Longer chain alcohols, tanins, and B vitamins are also present in all alcoholic beverages. Neither the alcohol itself nor these components represent a balanced source of nutrients.

The nutritional problems of the alcoholic are further compounded since time, money, and energy are deflected from the procurement of food. An alcoholic's diet is insufficient not only because of the empty calories consumed in the form of ethanol, but also because of poor appetite and inadequate food selection. Food that is ingested is poorly digested and absorbed. Alcohol causes direct inflammatory changes of gastric mucosa which modify the stomach's emptying and digestive processes. Active transport of the nutrients across the intestinal lining is also impaired, modifying the absorption of nutrients. In the liver, byproducts of ethanol oxidation alter the intermediate metabolism of proteins, vitamins, and hormones. Magnesium, zinc, and calcium deficiencies develop as a consequence of inadequate intake, and loss through vomiting, diarrhea, and increased urinary excretion. Similar mechanisms cause deficiencies of essential vitamins, particularly folic acid and thiamine. At the cellular level, ethanol also interferes with the utilization of vitamins and minerals that function as coenzymes and are important for fetal growth.

Metabolism of large quantities of ethanol within liver cells causes fat to accumulate which can predispose to alcoholic hepatitis and cirrhosis. Liver scarring in cirrhosis causes portal hypertension with esophageal varicies and ascities. Alcoholism is the most common cause of repeated attacks of pancreatitis. These can lead to chronic pancreatic insufficiency with subsequent nutritional deficiencies.

CARDIOVASCULAR SYSTEM

The direct effects of alcohol on the heart are dependent on the quantity and duration of exposure and must be separated from the effects of major associated risk factors such as smoking, nutrition, and lifestyle (Knott and Beard, 1982). Alcohol in high doses alters the function of the heart muscle through metabolic effects on lipids, proteins, carbohydrates, and minerals. Contractility and cardiac reserve are reduced. Heightened electrophysiologic excitability and increased conduction occur. However, acute exposure is not beneficial to coronary circulation since any hemodynamic changes are probably offset by metabolic consequences.

Metabolic changes and functional impairment precede morphologic alterations. Chronic heavy alcohol consumption can result in primary myocardial disease, including conduction disturbances. Drinking binges can produce transient arrythmias in individuals with no organic heart disease. Epidemiologic studies suggest that people who consume two drinks a day or less have a diminished incidence of myocardial infarction.

Alcohol also affects the peripheral circulatory system in a dose-dependent manner. Individuals consuming three or more drinks a day had higher systolic and diastolic pressures than did those having two or less drinks a day. Consumption of alcohol when disulfiram (Antabuse) is used can cause severe decreases in both systolic and disastolic pressure.

IMMUNE SYSTEM

Alcoholics are at increased risk of infection due to trauma, burns, and environmental exposure. The human immune system which normally provides protection from microbial infection is impaired by large quantities of alcohol. Cell-mediated immunity is hampered as alcohol decreases the ability of white blood cells to migrate to a site of infection. The macrophages' capacity to remove foreign substances also diminishes. A fall in the number of T-lymphocytes has been reported in alcoholics, and serum from alcoholics has been found to have inhibitory effects on lymphocyte transformations, necessary for cell-mediated immunity.

Humoral immunity also is impaired in alcoholics with cirrhosis. Although the number of immunoglobulins increase, there may be a decrease in their functional capacity. The cirrhotic liver has a reduced hepatic clearance of antigen–antibody complexes and bacteria due to a defective hepatic reticulo-endothelial system. The alcoholic is also particularly vulnerable to pneumonia because of impaired cilial function—the first line of defense in clearing inhaled particles from the tracheobronchial tree.

CENTRAL NERVOUS SYSTEM

Alcohol is consumed primarily because of its capacity to modify moods: low doses act as a stimulant while high doses are sedative.

It can be self-administered at a rate which will produce the amount of sedation and mood alteration that the individual desires. Subtle alterations in states of consciousness can be achieved by slowly sipping drinks. Individuals intent on altering memory and affect can drink at a rate which produces greater physiologic brain disruption. Under different circumstances alcohol may alleviate pain and anxiety, relieve inhibitions, or bolster illusions of power. Moderate doses cause reversible effects on neuronal membranes, temporarily altering the movement of ions and neurotransmitters and affecting the transmission of signals.

Chronic consumption of high doses of alcohol can irreversibly disrupt memory and judgment. Normal sleep and dreaming cycles are disrupted to varying degrees in different individuals, and the disruptions persist depending in part on dose and duration of exposure. Alterations have been observed in spontaneous and evoked neural activity. Alcoholics have an increased incidence of convulsions secondary to withdrawal and to head injuries resulting from accidents and violent incidents. Effects on the CNS are associated with pathologic changes in the neurophysiological functions and/or neuroanatomical structure of the brain. Physiologic changes at higher levels of the CNS can affect the hypothalamic area of the brain which in turn secretes releasing hormones that control anterior pituitary regulation of the endocrine system.

ENDOCRINE SYSTEM AND REPRODUCTIVE FUNCTION

In vertebrates, reproduction is under three levels of hormonal control. The first involves steroid hormones produced by the gonads: testosterone synthesized by the Leydig cells of the testis and estradiol and progesterone from the ovary. Steroids regulate development of the genitalia and the secondary sex characteristics. At a higher level, the structure and function of the ovary and testicle are regulated by gonadotropins secreted by the anterior lobe of the pituitary gland. This master endocrine gland produces ten different hormones which serve as messengers regulating the function of other glands. Among them are follicle stimulating hormone (FSH), luteinizing hormone (LH), prolactin, adrenocorticotropin (ACTH), and thyrotropin (TSH). Variations in the hormonal balance regulate the menstrual cycle, reproduction, and the internal physiology necessary for sustaining a successful pregnancy. At the third level, the anterior pituitary is regulated by the hypothalamus, which receives impulses from other centers in the brain. Several releasing factors from the hypothalamus are carried to the pituitary by a vascular connection. This neurovascular linkage integrates the functioning of the CNS and the endocrine system, and also provides feedback from the peripheral glands.

A fuller understanding of the effects of ethanol on the adult and the fetus has become possible with the development of new techniques for assaying minute amounts of hormones. Ethanol-induced alterations of the interaction between the CNS and the endocrine system change metabolic and reproductive functions. Chronic consumption of high doses of ethanol alters steroid synthesis, modifies pituitary function, and disrupts hypothalamic regulation.

In small doses, alcohol enhances sexual experiences for both sexes by inducing feelings of euphoria and relaxation. In contrast, acute intoxication limits sexual functioning. Chronic alcoholics are often passive and disinterested in sexual activities. Chronic male alcoholics demonstrate multiple disturbances in reproductive endocrinology and function. Impotence, decreased libido, testicular atrophy, infertility, proliferation of breast tissue, and loss of body hair are observed frequently. This feminization, once primarily attributed to the hyper-estrogenic state associated with Laennec's cirrhosis, has now been shown to also result from the direct effects of alcohol on the gonads and the hypothalamic-pituitary axis. From puberty until late adult life, millions of spermatazoa are produced daily in the testis. Spermatogenesis requires retinal (vitamin A), which is regenerated from retinol by alcohol dehydrogenase. When ethanol competes for the alcohol dehydrogenase, the testis becomes retinal-deficient and spermatogenesis decreases, despite an adequate amount of vitamin A in the diet. In addition, alcohol impairs the function of the Leydig cells which secrete testosterone. Decreased testosterone production has been observed following both a single acute dose and chronic ingestion of alcohol in humans and in experimental animals (Van Thiel and Gavaler, 1982). Changes were observed in testosterone levels at peak BACs of 109 mg percent (above the legal level of intoxication) (Mendelson, 1970a). Suppression of plasma testosterone was related to blood alcohol level, with the lowest levels of testosterone observed in association with the highest BACs. The drop in testicular levels of testosterone further reduces spermatogenesis and the volumes of the seminiferous tubules, producing gross testicular atrophy.

In women, heavy drinking has been shown to disrupt the menstrual cycle and decrease fertility (Mello, 1980; Cicero, 1980). Little is known about the mechanisms. Further research is necessary to differentiate disruption of the hypothalamic-pituitary axis from direct effects on the ovaries. Gonadotropin levels have not changed following the acute administration of high concentrations of alcohol (Mendelson, 1970b). However, the effects of chronic ethanol ingestion on hormone levels are difficult to evaluate because of the normal fluctuations that occur throughout the menstrual cycle.

Summary

Between 5% and 10% of pregnant women drink heavily, consuming far more than other pregnant women. Alcohol in high concentrations has the potential to adversely affect every maternal organ system and to disturb the maternal-placental-fetal system. Lower doses can alter moods but have no persistent effects. Of particular concern in pregnancy are changes in the liver and other parts of the gastrointestinal system, the immune system, the CNS, the cardiovascular system, and the endocrine and reproductive systems.

Three

Alcohol and the Fetus

Normal development represents an organized expression of genetically coded information with a high degree of resilience from generation to generation. The organizing force that controls the growth of complex structures in this reliable, repetitive fashion is not understood, but its power is clear from the fact that malformations are the exception rather than rule. The capacity of any teratogen to disrupt normal development varies throughout the growth process. Exposure at a sensitive stage may result in gross maldevelopment, even though each of the other steps takes place normally. An understanding of the stages of fetal development helps to explain alcohol's potential to cause a range of abnormalities. The information on fetal development reviewed in this chapter is adapted from Langman (1975) and Page et al (1976).

Organogenesis and fetal development

Fertilization of the mature egg occurs in the fallopian tube within 24 hours of ovulation. Between ovulation and fertilization the egg is vulnerable to chemical or environmental insults; exposure at this time probably would be lethal. During the 36 hours following fertilization, the first cleavage occurs. The egg then divides into two, four, eight, and sixteen cells, which form a solid ball. As cell division continues, a hollow ball, the blastocyst, develops and becomes implanted in the lining of the uterus about one week after fertilization. Following fertilization and before implantation the embryo is relatively resistant to damage (Hill, 1973). The blastocyst differentiates into structures which become the embryo and the early placenta. Between the second and the eighth week, through growth and differentiation, organ systems are established in an orderly sequence. From early differentiation through organogenesis, chemical disruption of the cellular membranes or metabolic functioning can markedly disturb development. Specific malformations depend on organ susceptibility at the time of exposure.

CENTRAL NERVOUS SYSTEM

Because of its complexity, the brain is the organ that grows most rapidly and develops over the longest period of time. At the beginning of the third week, the CNS is initiated as an elongated plate which forms raised folds. The folds then close over a depressed region—the neural groove—and fuse, forming a neural tube. The anterior aspect of the neural plate becomes the brain; the caudal regions form the spinal cord. As its size continues to increase, the anterior end of the neural tube bends downward, followed by a second flexure in a reverse direction. By the fourth week of gestation three primary brain vesicles have developed: forebrain, midbrain, and hindbrain. During the fifth week, cells from the lining of the neural tube divide repeatedly and migrate into adjacent layers, developing five regions of the brain. By the seventh week, two anterior-lateral bulges appear which will become the cerebral hemispheres. There is then an outward migration of neurones which form the cerebral cortex. The cerebellum begins to develop during the second month, and by the fourth month the cerebral hemispheres extend back to touch the cerebellar hemispheres. At this time the surface of the cerebral hemispheres is smooth, but during the latter half of pregnancy rapid growth causes the surface to become wrinkled and folded, forming gyrii. The period of rapid brain growth is characterized by active dendritic branching, synapse formation, and myelination.

Growth in utero is critical for the normal development of the CNS. The brain constitutes 12% of the body weight at birth (Dobbing, 1974). Brain weight doubles during the first year of life

and continues to grow rapidly, tripling in five years, at which time
it has reached 90% of its adult size. By adulthood the brain accounts
for only 2% of total body weight. This growth pattern differs from
that of the other organs, which continue to grow through adolescence. Most other body organs develop their basic structural organization by the third month of pregnancy; during the next two
trimesters fundamental changes are only in size and functional capacity.

GASTROINTESTINAL SYSTEM

The gastrointestinal system develops sequences of functions in utero
which enable it to absorb and metabolize the nutrients needed by
the infant. The small intestine is capable of peristalsis and of actively absorbing glucose by the 11th week of gestation, and as early
as the fourth month amniotic fluid is swallowed by the human fetus.
The liver begins to form by the third week; by the fifth week hepatic lobes are recognizable and the gall bladder has developed.
The fetal liver becomes capable of synthesizing protein and glycogen and of regulating blood sugar as well as synthesizing fetal hemoglobin and disposing of bilirubin. Glucose is provided by the
mother, with excess carbohydrate stored as glycogen in fetal liver,
muscle, and heart. Since the brain must be provided with glucose, a
malnourished fetus uses a considerably larger portion of his total
carbohydrate reserve to sustain cerebral function. In the normal
newborn, the brain is three times heavier than the liver; in the malnourished it may be seven or eight times heavier.
    Glycogen is first detected in the fetal liver at 10 weeks; by the
last third of pregnancy the carbohydrate content of the fetal liver
rises to twice the adult level. Glycogen is also stored in the skeletal
muscle and heart to provide energy during the birth period. Within
a few hours after birth glycogen values fall to adult levels. In malnourished infants, glycogen is depleted.
    The fetal liver also supplies enzymes for converting acetate to
fatty acids. The neonate may draw upon these fat reserves for calories during the first days of life. Liver enzyme activity changes
throughout pregnancy with the enzymes necessary for the metabolism of alcohol, alcohol dehydrogenase, and aldehyde dehydrogenase, developing late in pregnancy. In the neonate, they function

at a fraction of their adult capacity which is not attained until five years of age (Waltman et al, 1972; Cook, 1975).

RESPIRATORY SYSTEM

Around the 24th day of gestation the respiratory system begins developing as an outgrowth from the foregut. The bronchial tree takes form by a process of centrifugal branching, as the main bronchi repeatedly divide. By the end of the sixth month, 17 generations of subdivisions have been formed. An additional six divisions appear during postnatal life. Terminal air sacs or alveoli appear as outbranchings of the bronchioles. They are lined with flat epithelial cells which establish contact with capillary networks around the 28th week. At this point, the alveolar surface area and vascular portion of the lung are sufficient to permit a premature infant to survive. Prenatal preparation also requires development of chemical and neural controls, the carotid and corticopulmonary bodies. They are identifiable by the 60th day of gestation, although they do not regulate gas exchange until after delivery. At about 24 weeks' gestation, human alveolar cells start to produce surfactant, a surface-active agent which lowers surface tension at the air–fluid interface and prevents collapse of alveoli after birth.

Breathing movements in utero prepare the system for postnatal life but are not related to oxygenation, which is derived from the maternal system. Fetal breathing is episodic, occurring at about 30–70 breaths per minute, and is normally present about 65% of the time. Within a few seconds of birth, the respiratory system changes from a dormant, liquid-filled state to a system capable of breathing air.

ENDOCRINE SYSTEM

The fetal endocrine system also regulates functional organization. The first gland to appear is the thyroid. As early as the fourth week it can synthesize thyroglobulin, and by the tenth week it can accumulate iodine. By 12 weeks fetal triodo-thyronine and thyroxine regulate fetal metabolism. The fetal pancreas is differentiated by the third month and insulin is produced. Lypase is present in pancreatic sections by 16 weeks, and trypsin by 24 weeks, while amylase does not appear until several months after birth.

The fetal pituitary secretes ACTH by the tenth week and TSH by the 11th week. It is unlikely that maternal ACTH or TSH cross the placenta. Between the 12th and 20th week the fetal pituitary is secreting the gonadotropins, FSH and LH, which begin to regulate the fetal gonads. Steroids from the gonads regulate the developing CNS and play an important part in the sexual differentiation of the fetus. In the rat, abnormalities in the timing and peak of sexual hormone secretion in utero have been found to significantly alter adult sexual behavior (Anand and Van Thiel, 1982).

The placenta

The placenta is the organ that transfers nutrients and oxygen to the fetus and waste products of fetal metabolism (such as carbon dioxide and urea) to the mother's circulation. In the past, the placenta's role as a barrier was emphasized. Recently, however, it has become evident that most substances which circulate in the maternal blood reach the fetus. There are four known mechanisms for transport across the placenta. (1) Most small molecules, including oxygen and ethanol, move across the membrane by simple diffusion, propelled by the chemical gradient and not requiring additional energy. (2) Compounds such as glucose are transferred at a significantly more rapid rate than that of simple diffusion and probably utilize an additional transport system. (3) Amino acids move against a chemical gradient by means of an active transport system that requires energy. (4) Globulins, lipo-proteins, phospholipids, and other molecules too large for diffusion are moved across the placenta by pinocytosis in which the cellular membrane engulfs microdroplets.

A complex interplay of steroid production within the maternal-fetal-placental system sustains a critical balance throughout pregnancy by regulating the metabolism and physiology of the fetus and mother. The placenta manufactures chorionic gonadotropin and placental lactogen, hormones essential for maintenance of the pregnancy and growth of the fetus. It also synthesizes progesterone and other steroids which complement those produced by the mother and the fetus.

PLACENTAL SIZE

Normal placentae increase in size for up to 36 weeks. Restricted placental growth is associated with low birthweights and has been observed in association with malnutrition (Tremblay et al, 1965; Aherne and Dunnill, 1966). Kaminski et al (1976) observed that the average weight of placentae from 236 women who consumed over 1½ oz AA per day was 22 g less than that of 4,074 who drank smaller amounts of alcohol. When rats were exposed to acetaldehyde on gestational days 10, 11, and 12, growth of both the placenta and the umbilical cord was severely curtailed (Sreenathan et al, 1982).

MATERNAL-PLACENTAL-FETAL CIRCULATION
OF ALCOHOL

The uterine artery carries nutrients and oxygen to the placenta, where the circulation branches into the capillary bed and ultimately into chorionic villi. Diffusion occurs easily throughout pregnancy. During the later stages, the fetal and maternal circulation are separated only by the syncytiotrophoblast, a single mass in which individual cell membranes have disappeared, with a surface of approximately 11 square meters. Oxygen moves across it with an efficiency comparable to that in the lung.

Ethanol also diffuses easily across the placental membranes. Alcohol and acetaldehyde are small, nonionized molecules which are readily soluble in both lipids and water. While the placental barrier prevents the transfer of proteins and other macromolecules, small molecules pass through as if it were a sieve. The rate-limiting step is the rate of placental blood flow, not the rate of diffusion.

Alcohol crosses the placental membranes easily in both directions at a rate dependent on the concentration gradient. In 1900, Nicloux demonstrated that alcohol rapidly appears in the fetal circulation at concentrations similar to that in the maternal circulation. In more recent animal experiments ethanol labeled with radioactive carbon has been shown to distribute rapidly throughout the fetal body water (Ho et al, 1972; Åkesson, 1974).

Following ingestion of a single dose, the BAC of the mother will rise rapidly while the fetal BAC will lag behind. Maximum concentrations occur in the fetus many minutes later than in the mother

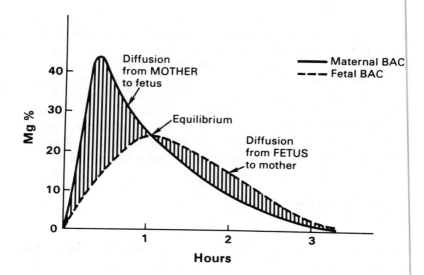

Fig. 3-1. Maternal and fetal BACs: diffusion of alcohol following a single drink.

and never reach as high a peak. As the mother metabolizes the alcohol, her BAC will drop. Since the fetal liver does not have mature ADH, the fetal BAC remains elevated until the maternal BAC falls (Seppälä et al, 1971; Idänpään-Heikkilä, 1972; Waltman et al, 1972). Then the alcohol will diffuse from the fetal circulation into the maternal circulation (see Fig. 3-1). Although the peak BAC reached by the fetus is lower, it is longer lasting than the mother's. When the mother drinks continuously and maintains a relatively steady BAC, an equilibrium develops between the maternal and fetal BAC and differences are small (Pratt, 1980).

Maternal and fetal levels of acetaldehyde have been difficult to determine. Early studies suggest that pregnant rats have higher blood acetaldehyde levels than nonpregnant rats following injection of 1.2 g/kg of ethanol (Kesäniemi, 1974). The elimination rate of ethanol was equal in pregnant and nonpregnant rats, but the acetaldehyde content of the peripheral blood after ethanol administration was higher in pregnant animals. Since no differences were found in the liver alcohol and aldehyde dehydrogenase, a difference in the extrahepatic metabolism of acetaldehyde was suggested. Pregnant mice were found to have lower acetaldehyde levels following treatment of 2.0 and 3.0 g/kg ethanol (Peterson et al, 1977). No differences were apparent with doses of 1.2 g/kg. Investigation of acetaldehyde levels in the fetus have also yielded inconsistent results. Randall et al (1977a) reported that acetaldehyde crosses the placenta and was detectable in fetal mice at 11 and 19 days. Kesäniemi and Sippel (1975) found no acetaldehyde in 22-day-old fetal rats, although levels in rat placentae were 25% of the maternal values. The inconsistencies may be due to dose responses, to greater placental oxidation of acetaldehyde in rats than in mice, to increased rate of placental oxidation during the third trimester, or to experimental problems of measurement. More reliable methods for determining blood acetaldehyde have recently been developed (Lindros, 1983). The reliability of future studies should improve with the incorporation of the new techniques.

If the mother is intoxicated at the time of delivery, the neonatal BAC is high. Newborns can have the odor of alcohol on their breath and be sedated. Since the enzymatic activity of the alcohol dehydrogenase in the newborn's liver is reduced, oxidation of ethanol occurs at a slower rate (Puschel and Seifert, 1979). Some alcohol is excreted in the newborn's urine and breath. When chronic maternal intoxication is sustained until the time of delivery both the maternal and fetal CNS develop tolerance. Withdrawal symptoms have been reported in infants born to chronic alcoholic mothers (these are considered further in Chapter 9).

Teratology

Teratology is the field of basic research that focuses on the causes of birth defects. Originally, teratologists described only gross structural defects in offspring. Now they investigate a range of consequences of in utero events: microscopic abnormalities, behavioral disorders, and biochemical consequences. Teratogenic agents seem to act in a specific way on a particular aspect of cell metabolism. They accentuate the incidence of defects which occur sporadically even in the absence of exposure. Malformations appear in a particular form because of underlying genetic instabilities.

Some teratogenic effects are obvious at birth; latent effects may not become apparent until the system becomes functionally mature or is challenged. The incidence of abnormalities varies with the age of testing, the technique of investigation, and the range of variability accepted as normal. Based on official records and birth certificates, the incidence of gross structural defects was between 0.75% and 1.98% (Langman, 1975). When hospital and clinic birth records were studied, the incidence noted was between 1.43% and 3.3%. Intensive examinations by groups of research pediatricians produced data which ranged from 2.2% in Germany to 8.76% in the United States. When children were examined at the end of one year, the rate doubled with the discovery of malformations which were difficult to identify in the neonate.

Until the early 1940s many thought that hereditary factors were the major cause of congenital defects. It was then discovered that children of women who had been infected with German measles virus during the early stages of pregnancy were at higher risk for eye, ear, and heart malformations. Subsequent research revealed that toxoplasma gondii and cytomegalovirus have teratogenic effects (Kalter and Warkany, 1983a). Other maternal illnesses, including diabetes, PKU, and vaginal bleeding, as well as environmental events such as exposure to X-rays, radium sources, and mercury are associated with fetal maldevelopment. A variety of drugs have been implicated in the development of abnormalities, thalidomide being the most dramatic example. The anticonvulsant drugs, including phenobarbital and diphenylhydantoin (dilantin), are associated with an incidence of major malformations similar to those of the FAS: heart abnormalities, microcephaly, and a characteristic facies. Administrations of hormones including synthetic progestins and cortisone also increase the incidence of anomalies. Deficiencies in vitamins and trace minerals such as zinc and magnesium are teratogenic in animals, however the effect in humans is less clear (Hurley, 1979). Various pesticides have also been suspected of being teratogenic, although, again, the evidence is clearer in animals than in humans.

All chemicals administered experimentally in sufficiently high doses retard the growth of some embryos or kill them (Kalter and Warkany, 1983b). Most embryotoxic agents have a threshold phenomenon which affords protection in many instances (Fabro, 1982). The timing of exposure also affects outcome. Exposure early in gestation causes morphologic damage or death; late in gestation, functional deficits and growth retardation occur (Wilson, 1973). In some instances, species resistance prevents the formation of lesions; in others, there is inclination for restitution. Restitution depends in part on the lesion's severity and timing. When the insult is severe or occurs late in gestation, remediation is not possible. In species with short gestational periods, restitution does not occur.

Even with this new understanding of multiple potential teratogens, the origin of most developmental defects remains unclear. Among all cases of mental retardation, approximately 90% are of unknown etiology. Similarly, the cause of most morphologic abnormalities is unexplained. Sokol (1981) has estimated that about 5% of all congenital anomalies may be attributed to prenatal alcohol exposure.

Adverse pregnancy outcomes

SPONTANEOUS ABORTIONS

Alcohol use during pregnancy has been associated with spontaneous abortion. Harlap and Shiono (1980) followed the pregnancies of 32,019 women to assess the incidence of spontaneous abortion. Questionnaires were administered at the first prenatal visit. In this population, 52% were nondrinking, 45% occasional drinkers (averaging less than one drink a day), and 2.9% were regular drinkers (averaging one or more drinks a day). Spontaneous abortions occurred among 1503 women (4.6%): 715 in the first trimester and 789 in the second. No effect of alcohol was observed on first trimester miscarriages. Of the 789 second trimester abortions, 37 occurred in women drinking 1–2 drinks a day and 12 among women reporting more than 3 drinks a day. A dose-response was demonstrated: the relative risk for occasional drinkers was 1.03, for women averaging 1–2 drinks a day it was 1.98, and for women reporting more than 3 drinks a day it was 3.53. When all drinkers were compared with nondrinkers, the relative risk was 1.10. Utilizing multiple regression analysis, alcohol and cigarettes were found to be independent risk factors; the effect of drinking was greater than that of smoking.

Kline et al (1980) compared the drinking patterns of 616 women who spontaneously aborted with those of 632 controls matched for age and hospital. In maximum-likelihood logistic regression analysis, alcohol use was associated with spontaneous abortion. The association persisted after control for several potentially confounding variables. The odds ratio for daily drinking was 2.58, for drinking twice weekly, 2.33. The authors conclude that frequency of drinking is consistently associated with spontaneous abortion provided that an average of at least 1 oz AA is consumed per occasion. Sokol et al (1980) also observed that the group of alcohol abusers was more than twice as likely to have a history of habitual spontaneous abortion. Larsson (1983) did not observe increased incidence of spontaneous abortions among the heavy drinkers nor were there differences in the number of previous miscarriages. An excess number of previous spontaneous abortions reported by the heavy drinkers at Boston City Hospital did not persist when differences in parity between the drinking groups were controlled (Weiner et al, 1983).

Experimentally, abortions have increased following alcohol exposure in monkeys (Altshuler and Shippenberg, 1981). Among rats and mice, alcohol has been associated with an increased rate of resorption (which is comparable to abortion in humans) in a dose-dependent manner (Chernoff, 1977; Randall et al, 1981; Persaud, 1983). The level of alcohol use which is implicated clinically is questionable. Comparing the studies of Kline et al (1980) and Harlap and Shiono (1980) with data from his study at a Cleveland hospital, Sokol (1980) observed that the risk was increased only for the heaviest drinking 2–4% of the women. He warns that quantitative data on drinking must be interpreted cautiously—that volumes and frequencies which appear to represent light or moderate drinking patterns may, in fact, due to denial, underreporting, and methods of calculation, represent heavy alcohol use. (A discussion of the problems of assessing alcohol use from self-reports appears in Chapter 7.)

Since it is likely that men who drink heavily mate with women who use alcohol, the role of paternal alcohol abuse in the incidence of spontaneous abortions should be investigated. A review of experimental research suggests that paternal alcohol abuse is associated with lethal mutations which cause abortions (Van Thiel and Gavaler, 1982) (see Chapter 9).

STILLBIRTHS

The association between alcohol use and incidence of stillbirth is unclear. Kaminski et al (1981) observed a statistically significant excess of stillbirths among the moderate/heavy drinkers in a study of 9236 women. The most frequent cause of death was abruptio placentae (Goujard et al, 1978). In two subsequent studies ($N = 3193$ and 1578), they observed an increased incidence of stillbirths among heavy drinkers, but the differences were not significant. The authors suggested that a low overall stillbirth rate and small sample size precluded detection of effects. In a sample of 200 pregnancies, Silva et al (1981) did not observe relationships between alcohol consumption and stillbirth. Sokol et al's (1980) prospective study of more than 12,000 pregnancies did not demonstrate an increased stillbirth rate or a history of more frequent induced abortion, stillbirths, and neonatal deaths among the alcohol group. If a large sample size (in excess of 9,000) is required to demonstrate the associations, then conclusions can not be drawn from prospective studies performed to date. A relationship is suggested by experimental data which has demonstrated an increased number of prenatal deaths in mice (Chernoff, 1977; Randall and Taylor, 1979), rats (Skosyreva, 1973) and beagle dogs (Ellis and Pick, 1980).

PREMATURITY

Alcohol's effects on the duration of pregnancy have been reported in several investigations of alcohol and pregnancy with inconclusive results. Prematurity was associated with alcohol consumption during pregnancy in two retrospective studies (Olegård et al, 1979; Kaminski et al, 1981) and with drinking prior to pregnancy in one (Hingson et al, 1982). No associations were found in four prospective studies representing more than 26,000 pregnancies (Sokol et al, 1980; Kaminski et al, 1981; Silva et al, 1981; Weiner et al, 1983), whereas a significant, but weak, relationship was noted in one (Tennes and Blackard, 1980).

In a study of possible risk factors for preterm delivery, Berkowitz (1981) observed that consumption of more than 7 drinks a week during pregnancy was associated with an increased risk of prematurity. Further analysis of 175 mothers and 313 matched controls demonstrated that the deleterious effects of alcohol on pregnancy maintenance were observed only among women drinking more than 14 drinks a week (Berkowitz et al, 1982). This dose-response or threshold effect may contribute to the inconsistent reports of the other studies.

Summary

Few teratogens have been as thoroughly investigated as ethanol. The multiple biochemical and pathophysiologic effects associated with ethanol and its metabolites have the potential to alter the growth and development of the embryo and fetus. A wide range of effects have occurred in children of women who drank heavily, either continuously or sporadically, during pregnancy. Animal studies have also shown structural, growth, and behavioral defects following maternal ethanol exposure to doses equivalent to 2 g/kg per day or more (Fabro, 1982).

Clinical and experimental evidence of the effect of in utero alcohol exposure on the developing fetus's growth, morphology, and CNS will be explored in the next three chapters.

Four

Growth

Growth retardation, both pre- and postnatal, is the most common anomaly associated with in utero exposure to alcohol. Failure to thrive was the clinical sign which initially brought children with fetal alcohol syndrome to the attention of Seattle researchers (Ulleland et al, 1970). Retarded growth is also associated with a number of other maternal risk factors, including age, parity, illness, malnutrition, cigarette smoking, licit and illicit drug use, and socioeconomic status (Miller and Merritt, 1979). Many of these risk factors are found more frequently among women who drink heavily during pregnancy (Weiner et al, 1983). The triad of the FAS (growth retardation, facial dysmorphology, and involvement of the CNS), however, identifies a subgroup of growth retarded infants with characteristics rarely found in association with other risk factors.

Among FAS children, either length is more profoundly affected than weight (Jones and Smith, 1973; Clarren and Smith, 1978), or length and weight are equally diminished (Lemoine et al, 1968; Dupuis et al, 1978). Both patterns differ from the effects of undernutrition alone, which affects weight more than length. Furthermore, growth retardation among severely affected FAS children persists even with adequate nutritional intake during hospital admissions and foster care placements (Lemoine et al, 1968; Hanson et al, 1976; Dupuis et al, 1978; Olegård et al, 1979; Majewski, 1981). In milder cases, growth retardation is less persistent, and some children reach normal size by maturity (Lemoine et al, 1968; Olegård et al, 1979).

Microcephaly is frequently observed among FAS children, occurring even after correction for small length and weight. Majewski (1981) reported that microcephaly becomes more apparent with increasing age. Its persistence into adulthood has been confirmed by radiographic evaluation (Smith et al, 1981). Small head circumference reflects small brain size and is often associated with CNS abnormalities. (See Chapter 6.)

The first case studies of FAS children described the most extreme manifestations of maternal alcohol abuse. Subsequently, the impact of a range of drinking patterns on fetal growth and development has been investigated in prospective and retrospective studies conducted throughout the world. Questions have been raised about the effects of heavy, moderate, and light drinking and about the effects of exposure during different gestational periods. Findings have varied. Some research groups have reported associations between intrauterine growth retardation and heavy drinking or alcohol abuse (Kaminski et al, 1976; Seidenberg and Majewski, 1978; Sokol et al, 1980; Silva et al, 1981; Kuzma and Sokol, 1982; Rosett et al, 1983b). Others report lower birthweights in association with moderate levels of drinking as well (Little, 1977). There are studies which show no association between alcohol consumption and fetal outcome (Tennes and Blackard, 1980; Hingson et al, 1982; Marbury et al, 1983). Some report that reduction of heavy drinking during pregnancy is associated with improved outcome on growth parameters (Olegård et al, 1977; Rosett et al, 1983b). In this chapter we review clinical research on alcohol consumption and growth, including our own findings at Boston City Hospital, and attempt to sort out the data. After discussing several studies, we shall try to explain the discrepancies between them in terms of methodological differences, and we will consider some animal studies which bear on the relationship between alcohol consumption and growth.

Epidemiologic research

Epidemiologic principles require that prospective studies use objective methods to obtain drinking histories and conduct neonatal examinations. Systematic testing procedures should be used. Interviewers should have no knowledge of neonate status, and examiners should not be aware of maternal drinking patterns. Confounding

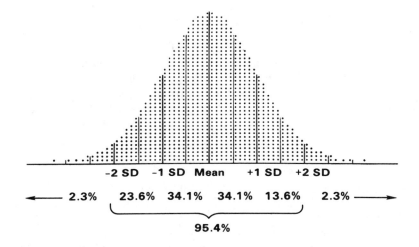

-2 SD   -1 SD   Mean   +1 SD   +2 SD

2.3%   23.6%   34.1%   34.1%   13.6%   2.3%

95.4%

Fig. 4-1. Normal distribution curve. (Reprinted with permission from Basic Books, Inc., Solomon Diamond, *Information and Error: An Introduction to Statistical Analysis,* Basic Books, Inc., New York, 1959, p. 82.)

variables must be considered and adequate controls included. The findings should be assessed for clinical as well as statistical relevance.

Before reviewing the studies, a brief description of the statistical terms that we will employ may be helpful. Statistical significance measures probability, demonstrating whether observed events are likely to occur by chance alone or are influenced by the variable being studied. The normal distribution of random events can be plotted as a bell-shaped curve (see Fig. 4-1). Standard deviation (SD) describes variation from the mean score. In a normal distribution, 1 SD represents the 68% of the population who score in the middle range; 2 SD includes an additional 27%, for a total of 95%. Measures which are more than 2 SD from the mean pertain to the 2.5% of the population with the lowest and highest scores, a small but highly significant portion of the population.

Significance levels are usually of interest when they are 0.05 or below. Significance at 0.05 states that there are five chances in 100 that the event would occur randomly; 0.001 represents one chance in 1000 of random occurrence. The lower the chance of random occurrence, the stronger the probability that there is a reproducible relationship between the variables.

Multiple regression analysis explores the impact of a set of possible predictors (independent variables) upon the outcome under study (dependent variable). Significant relationships mean that variance in the dependent variable can be accounted for by changes in the independent variables. Estimates can be made of the percent of change in outcome which can be accounted for by variation in each predictor.

THE PRENATAL STUDY AT BOSTON CITY HOSPITAL

At Boston City Hospital from 1974 to 1979 we studied patterns of alcohol consumption during pregnancy and their effects on the newborn. We found adverse outcomes among offspring of women who drank heavily throughout pregnancy, but no effects in association with rare or moderate drinking (Rosett et al, 1983b). Benefits were observed among newborns whose mothers reduced heavy drinking before the third trimester.

At the time of registration for prenatal care, we asked English-speaking women to participate voluntarily in a 15 minute structured interview designed to determine the volume and variability of alcohol intake, the use of other drugs, smoking, nutritional status, and demographic data. Cahalan's Quantity-Frequency-Variability Index was used to evaluate alcohol consumption (Cahalan et al, 1969). Separate questions were asked about the use of wine, beer, and liquor. Responses were standardized so that a "drink" represented the volume of beverage containing 15 cc (0.5 oz) of absolute alcohol, e.g., 360 cc (12 oz) of 4% beer, 120 cc (4·oz) of 12% wine, or 36 cc (1.2 oz) of 80 proof liquor.

Patients were classified as rare, moderate, or heavy drinkers, as defined in Chapter 2. Ten percent of the women reported heavy drinking: consuming more than 5 drinks on some occasions and at least 45 drinks per month. Women who reported drinking heavily were informed that they had a better chance of having a healthy baby if they abstained from alcohol use for the duration of their pregnancy. They were encouraged to participate in counselling sessions scheduled to coincide with their routine prenatal clinic appointments. (A detailed description of treatment strategies appears in Chapter 8.)

Data on maternal characteristics was collected consistently from May 1974 through September 1979. Infant evaluations were conducted in three cohorts. We approached each cohort with a somewhat different methodology. A pediatric neurologist examined the first cohort of 322 neonates (May 1974–June 1976). Growth data on a second cohort of 99 infants was abstracted from hospital records (June 1976–February 1977). In the third cohort, 469 newborns were examined by one of four pediatricians (February 1977–September 1979).

All pediatric examinations included neurologic and developmental evaluations and were administered in the newborn nursery by pediatricians with no prior knowledge of maternal drinking histories or any other information about the pregnancies. Length and head circumference were measured by the examining pediatrician. Weights were obtained from hospital charts. Gestational age was calculated using the Dubowitz score (Dubowitz et al, 1970). The Colorado Medical Center Classification of newborns was used to calculate growth percentiles (Lubchenco, 1976). Neonates with growth measurements at or below the tenth percentile were considered to be retarded, or small for gestational age (SGA).

In the first cohort of 322, 42 (13%) of the mothers were heavy drinkers: 128 (40%) were moderate drinkers; and 152 (47%) were rare drinkers (Ouellette et al, 1977). The heavy drinkers consumed an average of 5.8 oz AA per day; 31% of them drank between 8 and 16 oz AA per day. The mean daily dose was estimated at 2.2 grams of absolute alcohol per kilogram body weight.

Offspring of the heavily drinking women, as compared with offspring of the moderate and rare drinkers, demonstrated significantly more congenital malformations, growth retardation, and functional abnormalities ($p < 0.001$). Although these components of FAS were observed, the complete syndrome was not seen in any neonate. In later clinical observations, two cases of FAS were diagnosed. Signs that were ambiguous in the newborns were more definitive in older children.

Separate analysis was performed on offspring of women who drank heavily but had abstained or reduced their alcohol consumption before the third trimester (Rosett et al, 1978). Of the 15 infants born to reduced drinkers, 10 (67%) were normal, compared with only 2 (7%) of the 27 infants born to mothers who continued to drink heavily ($p < 0.001$).

In the second cohort of 99 infants, growth retardation was also observed among the offspring of 17 women who continued heavy drinking throughout pregnancy ($p < 0.001$) (Rosett et al, 1980). Ten women who reduced heavy drinking bore fewer babies with weight, length, or head circumference below the tenth percentile. Data on the 27 heavy drinkers in this cohort was combined with that of the 42 heavy drinkers in the first cohort for further analysis. Prenatal care alone did not improve prognosis; there were no significant differences between offspring of women who continued drinking heavily who did and did not receive prenatal care. When drinking patterns during the third trimester were held constant, potential confounding variables were found to have little effect on fetal growth. The percentage of growth retardation was consistently associated with maternal drinking and independent of smoking. No differences were found between offspring of heavy drinkers who abstained throughout pregnancy and those who reduced drinking to the moderate or rare range.

In a third cohort of 469 mother–infant pairs, heavy drinking was reported by 43 (9%), moderate drinking by 164 (35%), and rare drinking or abstinence by 262 (56%) (Rosett et al, 1983b). Mean daily absolute alcohol use reported by heavy drinkers (5.0 oz AA) was 15 times higher than that of the moderate drinkers (0.3 oz AA). The heavy drinkers differed statistically from the rest of the sample on several behavioral characteristics: they smoked more cigarettes, used more marijuana during pregnancy, and had had more experience with psychoactive drugs at some time in their lives. There were no differences between the women in ethnicity, parity, age, and mother's pre-pregnancy weight.

Several statistical techniques (chi-square, multiple regression, and matched pair analysis) demonstrated that heavy maternal alcohol consumption identified in the prenatal clinic and sustained throughout pregnancy was associated with a higher incidence of growth retardation and congenital abnormalities among neonates. This association was independent of eight other risk factors associated with growth in multiple regression analyses (Fig. 4-2). No differences were found between offspring of rare and moderate drinkers. Analysis of data on substance use revealed that the risk

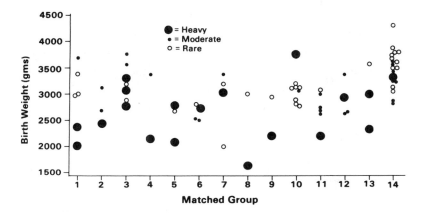

Fig. 4-2. Birthweights of neonates born to heavy drinkers and matched moderate and rare drinkers. *Large circles,* heavy drinkers; *small circles,* moderate drinkers; *open circles,* rare drinkers. Matching variables: parity, ethnicity, cigarettes, marijuana, mother's pre-pregnancy weight, mother's age, baby's sex, gestational age. (Reprinted with permission from the American College of Obstetricians and Gynecologists, *Obstet Gynecol* *61*(5):539–546, 1983.)

for growth retardation was related to alcohol use whether or not cigarettes or marijuana were used (Table 4-1). Findings on 469 mother–infant pairs in the third cohort were consistent with data from the first and second cohorts (Fig. 4-3).

Of the 43 women who reported drinking heavily at registration, 23 women participated in at least three counselling sessions in the prenatal clinic. Of these, 16 (69%) were judged to have abstained or significantly reduced their consumption below "heavy" levels before the third trimester. Two women who did not participate in counselling sessions reported reduced consumption and were considered reliable informants. Thus, there were 18 women who were judged to have markedly changed their drinking patterns—eleven abstaining and seven moderating their use. Women who reduced their consumption did not differ from those who sustained heavy drinking in the amount of alcohol they had consumed at the time of registration or in their sociodemographic characteristics. Neonates born to reduced drinkers were similar to offspring of the rare and

Table 4-1   Incidence of growth retardation in the prenatal study at Boston City Hospital

SUBSTANCE USE DURING PREGNANCY	BIRTHWEIGHT BELOW TENTH PERCENTILE FOR GESTATIONAL AGE
	N
A Sustained heavy drinking No cigarettes No marijuana	9/18 (50%)
B Sustained heavy drinking Used cigarettes and/or marijuana	10/34 (29%)
C No sustained heavy drinking Used cigarettes and/or marijuana	14/197 (7%)
D No sustained heavy drinking No cigarettes No marijuana	27/534 (5%)
Total population	60/783 (8%)

moderate drinkers in growth parameters, but they exhibited more congenital anomalies.

OTHER CLINICAL STUDIES

The relationship between heavy drinking or alcohol abuse and growth retardation has been observed in many studies (Table 4-2). Alcohol abuse was associated with increased risk for having an SGA infant among 12,000 pregnancies followed at a single hospital for a four year period (Sokol et al, 1980). Alcohol abuse was associated with other risk factors, including abuse of other drugs and cigarette smoking. Alcohol abuse and cigarette smoking each approximately doubled the risk of growth retardation. The risk of having an SGA baby was 1.8 for nonalcoholic smokers, 2.4 for alcoholic nonsmokers, and 3.9 for alcoholic smokers.

Associations between frequent beer drinking and low birthweight were demonstrated in an evaluation of 44 potential determinants of intrauterine growth among 5093 mother–infant pairs (Kuzma and

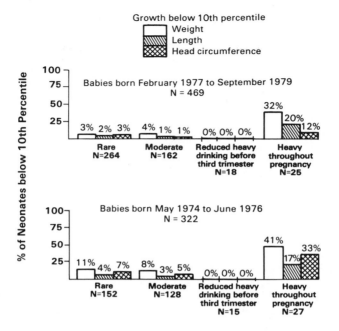

Fig. 4-3. Growth retardation by maternal drinking pattern in prenatal clinic at Boston City Hospital. (Reprinted with permission from the American College of Obstetricians and Gynecologists, *Obstet Gynecol* *61*(5):539–546, 1983.)

Sokol, 1982). Self-administered questionnaires were completed at the first prenatal visit by 63% of the study population and immediately postpartum by 37%. Separate questions were included on the frequency and quantity of beer, wine, and liquor consumption, as well as on the number and duration of heavy drinking occasions. Infant birthweight was adjusted for gestational age assessed by obstetric criteria. Utilizing regression analysis, absolute alcohol intake as an omnibus variable was not an important determinant of birthweight. However the frequency of beer drinking contributed independently to a reduction in birthweight: a decrement of 100 grams occurred among offspring of the 3% who drank beer most frequently. There were no differences between mean birthweights of children born to nondrinkers and children of women reporting less

Table 4-2   Patterns of alcohol consumption and neonatal growth retardation

	N	"HEAVY DRINKING"	"MODERATE DRINKING"
Sokol et al, 1980	12,000	+	−
Kuzma and Sokol, 1982	5,093	+	−
Rosett et al, 1983	322	+	−
	469	+	−
Silva et al, 1981	200	+	−
Kaminski et al, 1981	9,000	+	−
	3,200	−	−
	1,578	+	−
Marbury et al, 1983	12,440	NA	−
Gibson et al, 1983	7,301	NA	−
Hingson et al, 1982	1,690	NA	−
Tennes and Blackard, 1980	278	NA	−
Little, 1977	263	+	+

NA = Number of heavy drinkers identified too small for statistical analysis.

than 20 cans of beer per month following adjustment for caffeine and cigarettes. Curiously, frequency of wine drinking was correlated with increased birthweight. Wine and beer accounted for a very small portion (0.2%) of the total variance in weight.

Bottoms et al (1982) investigated fetal serum levels of thiocyanate (SCN), a component of beer and cigarette smoke. There was a direct correlation with the quantity of beer consumed and thiocyanate concentration after controlling for maternal characteristics, gestational age, and use of nicotine and marijuana. The relationships between thiocyanate level and fetal outcome have not been reported. The significance of nonethanol components of various beverages is an important subject for future investigation.

Alcohol's adverse effects on prenatal development were observed in the offspring of the heavy drinkers among 200 mother–infant pairs in Brazil (Silva et al, 1981). Women were classified as heavy drinkers if they reported daily or almost daily alcohol ingestion with at least five drinks on some occasions, or regular consumption of at least five drinks once a week. Nutritional parameters were not different between drinking groups. Infants of the heavy drinkers were small for gestational age, microcephalic, and had small palpebral fissures more often than infants born to moderate drinkers and abstainers.

Heavy drinking (more than 100 grams of alcohol a week) doubled the risk for having an SGA child among 900 infant–mother pairs (Wright et al, 1983). The risk was also increased by cigarette smoking. Among the 184 women who met the criteria for heavy drinking, 37 admitted to binges of more than 150 grams in a single session and 10 consumed more than 50 grams/day. Moderate drinking (less than 50 grams/week) did not increase the risk of having an SGA baby.

Birthweights were reduced among nine offspring of alcohol abusers as compared with 30 excessive drinkers and 360 occasional drinkers in Sweden, but the differences were not statistically significant (Larsson, 1983). Cigarette smoking was correlated with having an SGA baby. Marijuana use had a small, statistically insignificant effect on infant size. Infants of women who both drank abusively and smoked cigarettes had the lowest birthweight.

Inconsistent findings on the relationship between moderate/heavy drinking and low birthweights were reported in three cohorts of mother–infant pairs in France (Kaminski et al, 1981). Included in the study were 9000 births in the main public hospitals in Paris, 3200 births thought to be a representative sample for all of France, and 1578 births at one public hospital in Paris. Women were classified as non/light drinkers (< 400 ml AA per day, or three drinks) or moderate/heavy drinkers ($\geq$ 400 ml AA per day). The percentage of women defined as moderate/heavy drinkers in each cohort was 5.5%, 6.1%, and 1.6% respectively. Moderate/heavy drinking was associated with a lower mean birthweight of 58 g among offspring in the first cohort and 192 g in the third: no associations were found between birthweights and maternal drinking in the second cohort. No differences were observed in the characteristics of the women in each cohort which could explain the discrepant findings. One possible explanation is that alcohol's effects on weight are dose related and the dichotomy used in the analysis blurred differences between the effects of high and moderate drinking levels. Subdivision of moderate/heavy drinkers into two groups would have enabled the investigators to assess the separate effects. When outcome was compared according to type of beverage consumed, the 158 women (1.7%) in the first cohort who drank only beer were found to have smaller infants than the mothers who drank only wine, or wine and beer together. In the second cohort, although there were no differences in birthweight among drinking groups, infants born to beer drinkers were significantly smaller than those born to wine drinkers, light drinkers, or non-drinkers. Neither higher alcohol intake nor demographic characteristics explained this finding. No differences were found between infants born to women who drank up to three drinks a day and infants of abstainers.

Relationships between moderate alcohol consumption (an average of at least 1.0 oz AA per day) and low birthweight have been reported in one study (Little, 1977). A group of 263 women were interviewed in the fourth month of pregnancy about alcohol use in the six months prior to pregnancy (before) and the first four months of pregnancy (early). Data on drinking practices for the fifth through eighth months (late) was obtained in a second interview conducted in the eighth month. Sixty-four women reported moderate alcohol consumption before pregnancy, four of whom gave evidence of alcohol abuse. From before pregnancy to late pregnancy, the number of women reporting moderate consumption dropped to 20. Drinking in the moderate range before pregnancy was associated with a decrease in birth weight of 91 g; the same amount ingested in late pregnancy was associated with a decrease of 160 g. No relations were found for alcohol use early in pregnancy. The authors suggest that this lack of significance may be due in part to the small number of women with high AA scores in this period. Although women were defined as moderate drinkers, data on neonates born to the women who abused alcohol was not analyzed separately.

Opposite conclusions about moderate drinking were reached in other studies. Tennes and Blackard (1980) investigated the effects of socially prevalent drinking levels and found no association between drinking and birthweight among 278 mother–infant dyads. Women were interviewed three times: before 20 weeks gestation, at 6 or 7 months, and postpartum. Structured open-ended questionnaires were utilized to obtain information on dietary habits, use of licit and illicit substances, environmental hazards, and health status. Twenty percent of the sample were considered to be moderate drinkers, whose consumption ranged from one drink per week to 1½ drinks per day. Two percent were heavy drinkers averaging more than 1½ drinks per day. Using stepwise multiple regression analyses, separate calculations were made for alcohol use in early and late stages of pregnancy. Alcohol use was not significantly associated with neonatal outcome in any analysis. The authors concluded that moderate alcohol consumption had no effect on birthweight and that evaluation of heavy drinking was precluded by the small number of women reporting this drinking pattern.

A study of 1690 infant–mother pairs following delivery at Boston City Hospital revealed no associations between alcohol use and neonatal outcome (Hingson et al, 1982). Women were interviewed postpartum and information was collected on several maternal characteristics including drinking habits during pregnancy. Drinking more than 2 oz AA per day was reported by 2.8% of the women. Repeated multiple regression analyses were conducted using several drinking variables: frequency, usual quantity of consumption on drinking days, and average daily volume of beer, wine, and liquor. Alcohol use did not influence birthsize regardless of which measure was used. Heavy drinking was significantly associated with reduced birthweight among a subgroup of 328 neonates whose mothers had been interviewed in the prenatal clinic phase of the program. Significant associations between birthweight and the mother's weight, weight gain, race, age, illness, cigarettes, and marijuana use led the authors to suggest that other maternal habits may be more common than heavy alcohol use and may be more predictive of outcome.

In a similar study, alcohol consumption was not associated with low birthweight or congenital anomalies in 12,440 mother–infant pairs (Marbury et al, 1983). In this cohort, placenta abruptio was the only adverse outcome related to alcohol use when confounding variables were controlled in multiple regression analyses. Information on alcohol consumption during pregnancy was obtained in postpartum interviews. Alcohol use was coded as a dichotomous variable: women consuming 14 or more drinks per week ($N = 92$, 0.7%) were compared with all others. Consumption of more than 21 drinks per week was reported by 23 women. This small number of women decreases the power of the statistical techniques to detect differences associated with heavy drinking. Therefore, conclusions of this study pertain to moderate drinking.

Likewise, alcohol use was not associated with growth retardation or congenital anomalies among 7301 infants in Australia (Gibson et al, 1983). The authors state that the lack of association is a reflection of the very small number (1.5%) of women who reported heavy consumption. In this population, significant relationships were observed between cigarette smoking and infant size. Relationships were suggested between marijuana use and birthweights, but differences were not statistically significant.

The stage of pregnancy in which drinking occurs can affect outcome: third trimester exposure was associated with lower birthweights than was early exposure (Little, 1977). Improved outcomes have been observed following reduction of heavy drinking during pregnancy. As far back as 1899, Dr. William Sullivan, a prison physician in Liverpool, noted that alcoholic women who had previously borne sickly offspring had healthy children when forced by imprisonment to be abstinent. His observation has been confirmed in recent studies. In a retrospective study of 52 offspring of 15 alcoholic mothers, Olegård et al (1979) found that mean growth parameters at birth were 1 SD below national norms and mental retardation was prevalent. Children of five women who stopped drinking heavily between the 5th and 12th weeks of pregnancy had normal birthweights and ordinary school performance. Among another group of infants whose mothers reduced heavy alcohol use, birthweights were also normal (Hrbek et al, 1977; Hrbek et al, 1982). However, there was altered response to external stimuli (evoked response potentials), suggesting abnormal development of the central nervous system (see Chapter 6). Seidenberg and Majewski (1978) found fewer signs of alcohol embryopathy (AE) among offspring of women in chronic and crucial phases of alcoholism who reduced consumption during pregnancy. Seventy-two percent (18) of the heavy drinkers reduced their drinking. AE was diagnosed in 17% of the offspring of reduced drinkers as compared to 57% of those born to women who sustained heavy drinking. Wright et al (1983) reported no differences in birthweight when drinking was reduced before the fourteenth week of pregnancy. However, questions on reduction of alcohol use pertained to the one week prior to visiting the antenatal clinic (personal communication). No data is available on drinking patterns late in gestation. Further analysis of this data revealed that the risk of being SGA was 60% less for offspring of women who reduced drinking than for those who sustained heavy drinking (English and Bower, 1983).

Little et al (1980a) found differences in birthweights of infants of alcoholics who continued to drink throughout pregnancy (drinking), those who modified drinking patterns (abstinent), and controls. The sample included 100 recovered alcoholics recruited over an 18 month period through an extensive campaign of public announcements and personal contacts in two states (Little et al, 1979). Self-reports of alcohol consumption during the target pregnancy were obtained during interviews conducted an average of 7½ years after the pregnancy. Compared to controls, the mean birthweight was 493 grams lower among offspring of the continuously drinking women and 258 grams lower in the abstinent alcoholic group. Statistically significant differences occurred between mean birthweights in the three groups: continued and controls ($p < 0.001$), abstinent and controls ($p < 0.05$), abstinent and continued ($p < 0.05$).

Case reports as well as retrospective and prospective studies offer clear demonstrations of the adverse effects on fetal growth of exposure to high doses of alcohol throughout pregnancy. The effects of lower doses and of reducing drinking during pregnancy seem controversial. However, many of the differences between the findings on the relationship between alcohol and growth result from research techniques. An understanding of methodologic issues helps to bring about convergence between the findings of the several studies.

LIMITATIONS OF STUDY DESIGNS

Growth would seem to be an easily standardized variable since there are instruments for measurement and charts to evaluate weight, length, and head circumference. However, measurements can vary with research protocols and examiner differences. While standard nursery scales can determine weight with great accuracy, timing is important. Since there is a weight loss during the first few days postpartum, infants should be weighed almost immediately after birth. It is difficult to reliably measure length since infants tend to flex into a fetal position. To help overcome this flexed position, some examiners use the tonic neck reflex. Several devices are available that improve the reliability of length measurements (Miller and Merrit, 1979). Few FAS studies have described the methods that were used to validate length measurements. Head circumference should be measured along the occipital frontal axis and excessive tension on the tape avoided.

Assessment of neonatal size, to be valid, should include consideration of gestational age. Decrements of 100–200 grams from a mean birthweight can be caused by a myriad of factors and have little clinical relevance (Lubchenco, 1976). The categorization of an SGA infant is based on a standardized examination of gestational age (e.g., Dubowitz) and a classification of weights for gestational age (e.g., Lubchenco). A weight which is below the tenth percentile for age reflects growth retardation and is considered to have clinical implications, marking infants at risk for morbidity and mortality. When studies utilized SGA as the measure of growth retardation, heavy drinking was associated with neonatal size while moderate drinking was not (Rosett et al, 1983b; Ouellette et al, 1977; Silva et al, 1981; Sokol et al, 1980). An association between moderate drinking and infant size was observed only when growth retardation was measured as decrements from mean birthweights without adjusting for gestational age (Little, 1977).

The lack of standardized terms for drinking patterns makes it difficult to compare the results of separate studies. Each investigator has independently defined drinking patterns in the study population. The heaviest drinking group of women within each population has been variously labelled as heavy (Kuzma and Kissinger, 1981; Sokol et al, 1981; Rosett et al, 1983b), moderate/heavy (Kaminski et al, 1981), heavy social (Fried et al, 1980), moderate (Little, 1977), and social (Harlap and Shiono, 1980). In each study, regardless of the label, alcohol was related to adverse outcome only among women whose drinking patterns were in the top 10% and most often in the top 5%, suggesting a dose-response or threshold effect.

In the three studies that did not observe relationships between drinking and birthweight, the small number of heavy drinkers precluded assessing the impact of this level of drinking through the statistical technique of regression analysis (Tennes and Blackard, 1980; Hingson et al, 1982; Marbury et al, 1983). Therefore, their findings pertain only to moderate or rare drinkers and support the hypothesis that there is a dose-response or threshold effect, rather than a linear relationship between alcohol consumption and birthweight.

Women have been divided into drinking groups according to minimum averages of consumption, and outcomes have been attributed to the lowest doses. Ranges and means of drinking which more accurately describe actual consumption demonstrate high levels of use within these groups. Kuzma and Kissinger (1981) reported mean alcohol consumption of 5.9 oz AA per day among a group of women drinking 2 oz or more per day. Similarly, a mean of 4.6 oz AA per day occurred in a group of women whose daily average was at least 0.75 oz per day with 5 drinks on some occasions (Rosett et al, 1978). Many studies have not provided information on means and ranges. Growth retardation may be associated with the higher levels of use within the group and falsely attributed to the lowest.

Precise measurements of alcohol use are difficult to obtain when relying on self-reports (see Chapter 7). Alcohol intake reported in surveys of the general population is estimated to be 50% less than the quantity of alcohol sold (Fitzgerald and Mulford, 1978). It is likely that amounts reported by pregnant women and new mothers are far lower than the amounts actually consumed. The difficulty of obtaining accurate information about alcohol intake during pregnancy is compounded in retrospective studies. Underreporting is clear for a subgroup of the 1690 women interviewed postpartum at Boston City Hospital. Interviews had been conducted in the prenatal clinic with 328 of these women. For this subgroup, heavy alcohol consumption, whether measured prenatally or postpartum, was associated with a significant decrement in birthweight. During the prenatal interview, 10.7% of these women had reported drinking heavily, whereas in the postpartum interview only 3.6% reported drinking heavily during pregnancy (Alpert et al, 1981). Among 1362 women who were interviewed only in the hospital, 1.7% reported heavy drinking. Since the two groups did not differ significantly on sociodemographic variables it is likely that underreporting was at least as great among the 1362 who were interviewed only postpartum. Miscategorization of heavy drinkers may have masked the relationship between heavy drinking and fetal development and led to the conclusion that other factors were more prevalent and more important.

The relationship between low birthweight and maternal alcohol use has been reported to be stronger for consumption in late pregnancy than in early pregnancy (Little, 1977; Olegård et al, 1979; Rosett et al, 1983b). Animal experiments have also demonstrated that fetal exposure during the third trimester has the greatest impact on birthweight (Abel, 1979b; Lochry et al, 1982). Examination of third trimester drinking patterns separately from first and second trimester shows a marked reduction in consumption levels during pregnancy (Little, 1977; Fried et al, 1980; Tennes and Blackard, 1980; Sokol et al, 1981; Weiner et al, 1983). Therefore, an analysis of neonatal data which does not consider gestational stage of maternal alcohol ingestion may show weaker measurements of the adverse effects of heavy drinking and may miss the benefits of reduction.

Experimental research

Important issues that remain unresolved in clinical and epidemiological studies are questions concerning the dose and timing that
produce adverse fetal effects. Is there a standard dose-response
curve with a threshold or does alcohol have adverse effects at the
lowest concentrations measurable? Are adverse effects only incurred
by women who drink throughout pregnancy? Can a single binge at
a critical stage of gestation irreversibly damage the fetus? Can abstinence late in pregnancy mediate damage incurred in the early
stages? With experimental models these issues can be investigated
by administering precise doses, carefully monitoring blood alcohol
concentrations, and controlling gestational stage of exposure.

Also unanswered is whether alcohol itself is teratogenic or if
maldevelopment is due to associated risk factors. Fetal growth is
affected adversely by multiple factors, including maternal age, nutrition, smoking, other drug use, parity, and stress. Since in humans
many of these risk factors are associated with one another and with
alcohol use, it is difficult to isolate the individual effect of each risk
factor, even with large populations and multiple regression techniques. In the animal model, these risks can be studied individually
and in combination to isolate specific and synergistic mechanisms.

Animal researchers use a variety of techniques which could
never be used clinically for ethical reasons. The effects of alcohol
alone can be investigated in embryos growing in vitro. In vivo animal pregnancies can be terminated at various stages, and specific
modifications in organ structure and cell size can be evaluated se-
quentially. Access is available to organs such as the central nervous
system which can only be studied in humans following death.

Animal experiments must be evaluated carefully if they are to
have clinical relevance. There are advantages to using different
species, depending on the research question under study. Changes
that are observed may be species-specific, caused by genetic and
biochemical characteristics. Differences in length of gestation, developmental stages, and litter size must be considered. The route of
alcohol administration affects blood alcohol levels, nutritional status,
and stress levels. Caution must be taken in comparing doses in animal studies because of the wide variations in the rate of metabolism.
Animals must be given much higher doses than humans to achieve

similar blood alcohol levels. Procedural considerations in experimental research are discussed further in Chapter 7.

In animal studies just as in human studies, lowered birthweights have been the most consistently observed and dramatic effect of in utero alcohol exposure (Randall, 1982). Decreased intrauterine and postnatal weights have been reported in offspring of all animal species studied, including mice (Randall et al, 1981), rats (Abel, 1979b), beagle dogs (Ellis and Pick, 1980), miniature swine (Dexter et al, 1980), monkeys (Altshuler and Shippenberg, 1981), and sheep (Potter et al, 1980).

DOSE RESPONSE

Ethanol's effect on intrauterine growth has been shown to be dose related. In studies using inbred strains of mice, oral administration of ethanol prior to mating and throughout gestation revealed a definite growth deficiency due to alcohol in a dose-dependent manner (Chernoff, 1977; Randall et al, 1981). In rats, intraperitoneal administration of high doses of alcohol was related to weight reduction, while low doses were not (Anders and Persaud, 1980). Embryotoxic effects of alcohol were observed in rats in vitro only when alcohol concentrations reached those found in intoxicated humans, and they increased in direct relation to alcohol concentrations (Skosyreva, 1973). Doses of 1–2 g/kg/day produced BACs of less than 150 mg percent and had little effect on birthweights in rats and dogs (Abel, 1978; Ellis and Pick, 1980). Minimal effects on birthweights and growth patterns of rats pups exposed to 1–2 g/kg/day were attributed to decreased food intake rather than to ethanol. Significant growth retardation occurred with doses of 4 g/kg/day (BAC of 150–200 mg percent) (Abel and Dintcheff, 1978). However, animals exposed to 4 g/kg/day demonstrated catch-up growth by day 21 postpartum, while permanent growth retardation occurred in rats and dogs exposed to 6 g/kg/day (BAC of 200–270 mgs percent) (Abel, 1979a; Ellis and Pick, 1980).

GESTATIONAL STAGE

Growth retardation is dependent on gestational stage at time of exposure to alcohol. The degree of fetal growth retardation associated with alcohol administered in the third week alone was similar to retardation caused by alcohol administered throughout gestation (Abel, 1979b). Exposure in weeks 1 and 2 had lesser effects on birthweights. Lochry et al (1982) reported that C3H mice exposed to a single alcohol dose on gestational day 18 had lower birthweights. Body weight decreased as alcohol dose was increased from 2.5 to 5.0 g/kg. Weight reductions in mice exposed in the early stages of pregnancy were not so great.

GENETIC SUSCEPTIBILITY

Susceptibility to alcohol's effects on growth and morphology depends, in part, on genotype. An early mouse model of FAS demonstrated that the strain with lower ADH activity was more sensitive to ethanol than the strain with the greater metabolic capacity (Chernoff, 1977). Decreased birthweights were observed among DBA mice but not among C57BL given similar doses (Yanai and Ginsburg, 1977). Human variability in genetic vulnerability was observed in a pair of fraternal twins born to a mother who had consumed at least one quart of red wine and an unspecified amount of hard liquor daily throughout pregnancy (Christoffel and Salafsky, 1975). Although both boys showed signs of FAS, one's growth parameters were more markedly affected: weight, length, and head circumference were at or below the 10th percentile. The weight of the twin brother was at the 30th percentile, length at the 15th percentile, and head circumference at the 60th percentile. Both showed facial characteristics of FAS and both were jittery. Both were retarded in postnatal growth and development. Santolaya et al (1978) also reported a set of fraternal twins in which one was more severely affected. In one set of identical twins born to a chronic alcoholic, both offspring were affected with marked similarity in dysmorphology and growth (Palmer et al, 1974). Individual genetic differences in fetal susceptibility and maternal metabolic capacity may explain why some women who drink heavily throughout pregnancy have severely affected children while others drink similar quantities and do not (see Chapter 5). Vulnerability may also be related to the placenta's location within the uterus and the available blood supply of that area of the endometrium.

DIRECT EFFECTS OF ALCOHOL

Experimental replication of growth retardation demonstrates the direct effects of alcohol independent of confounding factors. In vitro exposure of rat embryos to 150 or 300 mg percent alcohol caused a decrease in total cell count as well as decreased crown–rump and head lengths (Brown et al, 1979). Acetaldehyde, the first metabolite of alcohol, has also been shown to independently retard growth and development (O'Shea and Kaufman, 1979; Popov et al, 1981; Sreenathan et al, 1982). Exposure to ethanol and to ethanol and nicotine combined demonstrated significant and similar effects on weights of fetal rats (Abel et al, 1979; Persaud, 1982). Prenatal exposure to nicotine alone had no effects. The experimental technique of pair-feeding has shown that restricted caloric intake alone did not cause growth retardation (Randall et al, 1981). Alterations in fetal body composition and electrolyte content observed in rat pups were considered to be specific to alcohol exposure (Abel and Greizerstein, 1979). Fetal whole body water and sodium content increased while lipid-free solid content decreased. These results can not be attributed to the restricted diet since the controls were pair-fed. In addition, the changes are not consistent with those commonly found with malnutrition. Significant variability in weight and length of individual fetuses within the alcohol group further suggests that not all offspring are similarly affected.

POSTNATAL GROWTH RETARDATION

Postnatal growth retardation persists in rats despite fostering to nonalcoholic dams and ad libitum access to food (Abel, 1979b). Abel (1981a) has demonstrated that retarded postnatal growth is not due to metabolic changes in utilization of food. Nor is it secondary to intestinal protein malabsorption; intestinal weights were similar for rats chronically exposed in utero to alcohol and for pair-fed controls (Ghishan et al, 1981). Intestinal transport of amino acids was also unaltered in the alcohol-exposed rat pups.

Disturbances in growth hormones have been observed in association with growth retardation in the rat (Thadani and Schanberg, 1979). However, endocrinological studies of children of alcoholics have demonstrated appropriate levels of growth hormone, thyroid hormone, cortisol, and gonadotropins. An analysis of hypothalamic-pituitary function in four children aged 9–15 who were born to an alcoholic woman demonstrated normal biochemical and endocrine test values (Root et al, 1975). Human growth hormone secretion was assessed in five FAS children after insulin-induced hypoglycemia and on a separate day after arginine infusion (Tze et al, 1976). The response was a normal or slightly hypernormal level of growth hormone and normal somatomedin activity. Investigation of thyroid function, creatinine, calcium phosphorus, 17-ketosteroids, and 17-corticosteroids in eight FAS patients revealed no abnormalities (Spiegal et al, 1979). However, peripheral unresponsiveness to growth promoting hormones may be a causative factor in the persistence of growth retardation (Castells et al, 1981).

Summary

Prenatal growth retardation has been consistently observed clinically and experimentally following exposure to high doses of alcohol. In some instances, growth retardation persists despite vigorous therapeutic strategies. The extent of the retardation is dependent primarily on dose and gestational stage of alcohol consumption and to a lesser extent on genetic susceptibility. Compensatory growth has been observed when in utero exposure to high doses has ceased. There are undoubtedly multiple mechanisms which can disrupt fetal growth. In vitro studies indicate direct effects of alcohol and acetaldehyde on cell differentiation and growth (Brown et al, 1979; Popov et al, 1981). Retarded growth can be caused by chronic fetal hypoxia (Abel, 1982a), hypoglycemia (Tanaka et al, 1982b), or hypothermia (Henderson et al, 1980), all of which have been experimentally produced by alcohol. Chronic exposure can interfere with the passage of amino acids across the placenta (Henderson et al, 1981; Fisher et al, 1982) and with the incorporation of amino acids into proteins (Henderson et al, 1979). Probable mechanisms are discussed more fully in Chapter 5.

Five

Morphology

Alcohol, like other teratogenic agents, is associated with a spectrum of malformations related to dose and timing. The multiplicity of effects suggests that alcohol can alter development throughout gestation. Case reports of FAS patients have noted abnormalities involving almost every organ system. Some epidemiological studies have reported a small but statistically significant increase in the incidence of morphologic abnormalities among the children of heavy drinkers (Ouellette et al, 1977; Hanson et al, 1978; Sokol et al, 1980; Rosett et al, 1983b). However, neither case reports nor epidemiologic studies demonstrate a unique and consistent pattern of associated anomalies other than the signs of FAS. Since these anomalies are nonspecific and occur in the general population, it is difficult to establish alcohol's causal role and to ascertain incidence rates.

From a review of 65 of their own cases of FAS and 180 from the world literature, Clarren and Smith (1978) classified associated abnormalities as principal ($> 50\%$), frequent ($> 25\%$), and occasional ($> 1\%$). Since the frequencies were derived from cases reported by different specialists in different countries, there was no standardization of criteria or examinations. Those which were observed frequently are of concern, those seen rarely should be evaluated with caution. Additional case reports confirm observations that alcohol affects the heart, face, genitalia, liver, skeleton, muscles, kidney, skin, brain, and immune system. It has also been associated with tumors in several FAS children.

Morphologic abnormalities that have been reported in association with alcohol abuse are described below. All have occurred in patients diagnosed as FAS. In all instances the magnitude of the anomaly correlated with the severity of the primary diagnostic criteria of FAS. (Alcohol's effects on the CNS are discussed in Chapter 6.)

Because of the number of associated birth defects, complete periodic physical examinations and relevant diagnostic procedures are indicated for FAS children. In the absence of a thorough examination, some dysmorphology may not become apparent until early childhood. Other anomalies may remain asymptomatic. Early identification and treatment of some malformations, such as those of the cardiovascular, genitourinary and ocular systems, can prevent later complications.

Abnormalities

OCULAR

Abnormalities that commonly occur in the eyelids and other periocular structures include short palpebral fissures, epicanthal folds, ptosis, strabismus, and blepharophimosis. Since there is great variation in the shape of the face and head associated with ethnicity and familial differences, these features must be carefully evaluated.

Short palpebral fissures were observed in 35 of 38 FAS patients in Seattle and were considered to be the most consistent physical feature of the FAS (Hanson et al, 1976). However, retrospective and prospective studies have not confirmed the association between palpebral fissure size and alcohol consumption (Majewski, 1981; Dooling, personal communication). In later reports Clarren (1981) stated that frank micro-opthalmia has been rare and that other abnormalities are more common. Methodologic difficulties may contribute to inconsistencies in reports on palpebral fissure size. To be standard, measurements should be adjusted for gestational age and ethnicity, but few norms are available (Jones et al, 1978). Measurement of palpebral fissures is best accomplished with a transparent ruler held in front of each eye across the longest horizontal axis. The infant must be relaxed with eyes spontaneously open. Since the eye is spherical and the ruler must be held at a distance in front of the plane of the fissure, a parallax error is inevitable. Interjudge reliability is poor: at Boston City Hospital, mean palpebral fissure widths varied from 18.3–20.1 mm between four examiners ($p < 0.001$).

Ophthamologic examinations have revealed intraocular anomalies which were not previously apparent, including optic nerve hypoplasia or atrophy and tortuosity of the retinal vessels (Rabinowicz, 1980). Among 21 children diagnosed as FAS, Stromland (1981) found optic disc hypoplasia and malformations of the retinal vessels in eight. Changes in retinal vasculature and steepness of the corneal curvature were observed in 17 Indian children (Garber, 1982). High astigmatism occurred in more than half of these cases, an incidence rate greater than that of the general Indian population.

ORAL

Among FAS children, observations have been made of prominent lateral ridges, cleft lips and palates, and small teeth lacking enamel (Clarren and Smith, 1978). Oral motor delays with feeding deficiencies were evident in three FAS infants (Van Dyke et al, 1982). Oral reflexes were normal but suck patterns were limited, with little ability to sustain more than two sucks. In prospective studies, poor sucking among offspring of heavy drinkers was clinically observed by Ouellette et al (1977) and measured with a pressure gauge by Martin et al (1979). Experimental studies corroborate these findings (Chen et al, 1982). Rat pups whose mothers had been fed liquid diets containing 35% ethanol-derived calories demonstrated a delay in nipple attachment, which lessened with maturity.

Tracheal intubation in conjunction with administration of anesthesia to two FAS children proved to be extremely difficult (Finucane, 1980). The problems were unanticipated since on external examination the airways did not appear to be abnormal.

OTOLOGIC

Deafness has been observed in four FAS children (Flint, 1983; Grundfast, 1983). In addition to these case reports, abnormal responses to somatosensory stimuli in both clinical and experimental studies have been reported (Hrbek et al, 1982; Church and Holloway, 1980). Hearing loss may contribute to learning problems and language dysfunction, which are discussed in Chapter 6.

SKELETAL

Associated skeletal abnormalities include radioulnar synostosis, hypoplastic toenails, shortened fingers, camptodactyly of fingers, clinodactyly of toes, flexion contractures of the elbow, pectus excavatum, hemivertebrae, and scoliosis (Clarren and Smith, 1978). Radiologic review revealed multiple findings in each of 12 FAS children, aged 5–12 (Cremin and Jaffer, 1981). In general, the features were nonspecific, reflecting the clinical condition of retarded growth. Congenital fusion of two or more cervical vertebrae was observed in X-rays of 19 of 38 severe FAS cases, ranging in age from 4 months to 17 years (Tredwell et al, 1982).

Radioulnar synostosis in which the proximal end of the radius is fused with the ulna has been noted in several independent reports. Bilateral absence of the radial heads and radioulnar synostosis were reported in a single case (Hayden and Nelson, 1978). Primary radioulnar synostosis occurred bilaterally in 4 of 8 FAS cases (Spiegal et al, 1979). Radiographic studies of 3 adults and 12 children ranging in age from 5–16 years revealed radioulnar synostosis and carpal fusion in three (Jaffer et al, 1981; Cremin and Jaffer, 1981). These uncommon anomalies were previously thought to occur sporadically as familial traits unrelated to alcohol exposure.

CARDIAC

Atrial and ventricular septal defects ranging from mild to severe are the most common associated cardiac pathology. Among 50 FAS children with cardiac anomalies, Dupuis et al (1978) reported 12 ventricular septal defects for which surgery was indicated, 12 interatrial septal defects which were well tolerated, and 25 small or medium ventricular septal defects with no potential for exacerbation. Among 56 FAS children with lesions, Loser and Majewski (1977) observed 10 atrial septal defects, two ventricular septal defects, and four other malformations. Sandor et al (1981) reported cardiac pathology in 31 of 76 (41%) FAS children ranging from newborn to 18 years of age; ventricular septal defects were the most common lesions, with tetralogy of Fallot and secundum atrial septal defects occurring less frequently. An additional 12 (16%) had functional murmurs. Noonan (1976) also reported an FAS case with tetralogy of Fallot. Patent ductus arteriosis and pulmonary artery dysplasia have been reported by others (Steeg and Woolf, 1979). The majority of lesions respond well to medical management, including those which have required surgery.

The incidence of cardiac defects, initially estimated at 50% (Hanson et al, 1976), has been found to vary with the severity of the FAS. Loser and Majewski (1977) found cardiac malformations in 29% (16/56) of all cases. Among those with the most severe facial dysmorphology and growth retardation, 59% were affected, while 5% of the mildly affected demonstrated cardiopathies. An incidence of 30% (14/47) was observed by Dehaene (1977b), who suggested that the "cardiac risk" was actually between 10% and 20% since the cardiopathies were small ventricular defects with little clinical significance.

RENAL

A spectrum of anomalies of the kidney and urinary tract has been observed among children with moderate or extensive signs of FAS. Malformations cited in eight case reports include hydronephrosis (Tenbrinck and Buchin, 1975; Hanson et al, 1976), fused ectopia, renal hypoplasia with obstruction of ureteropelvic junction (Goetzman et al, 1975), renal hypoplasia and urogenital sinus (Ijaiya et al, 1976), renal hypoplasia (De Beukelaer et al, 1977), and obstruction of ureteropelvic junction (Goldstein and Arulanantham, 1978).

Urologic examinations of 26 FAS children demonstrated malformations in nine cases (Havers et al, 1980). The anomalies were heterogeneous, ranging in severity from clinically insignificant to those requiring surgical intervention. They included single hypertrophied kidney, pyelonephritis, bilateral megaloureteral duplication and hydronephrosis, hypoplastic kidney with hamartomas and hydroureter, bladder diverticula, double collecting system, urogenital sinus, vesico-vaginal fistula, and caliceal cyst. Three of the malformations were observed in children who had exhibited no urological symptoms. Abnormal variations in kidney length and extremely bifid renal pelvis were found in two patients but were considered to be of little significance. Developmental abnormalities of the kidney were found in six additional FAS patients (Qazi et al, 1979). Although renal pathology was not of the same type in each case, four had either unilateral or bilateral renal hypoplasia.

Most studies of children with FAS do not include routine renal evaluations by radiologic or ultrasonic methods. Since many of the reported cases have been asymptomatic, incidence rates are impossible to estimate. When FAS children present any clinical or laboratory evidence of urinary tract disease a thorough work-up is indicated. Early diagnosis and correction of anomalies can reduce further urinary tract infections, urolithiasis, obstructions, acidosis, and uremia, all of which can contribute to growth retardation and severe morbidity.

HEPATIC

Hepatic disease has been observed in several FAS cases. Habbick et al (1979) reported three cases of FAS with liver abnormalities. Thick sclerotic central veins were observed in two patients, one of whom had symptoms typical of congenital hepatic fibrosis and cystic disease of the kidneys. In a third, liver abnormalities were thought to be secondary to cardiovascular problems which ultimately caused the infant's death. Møller et al (1979) observed liver disease with moderate bile duct proliferation in a single case of FAS. The small tubular structures in the portal spaces were characteristic of adult cirrhotic liver tissue. Symptoms of liver disease disappeared by 2 years. In another case report, light microscopic and ultrastructural hepatic changes characteristic of liver disease seen in adult alcoholics were observed in a 17-month-old FAS child (Lefkowitch et al, 1983). At age 4½, serum transaminases were essentially normal.

Newman et al (1979) described the simultaneous occurrence of extrahepatic biliary atresia (EBA) and FAS. At five years of age the patient had cirrhosis, hyperbilirubinemia, and rickets. Since EBA is uncommon, with an estimated incidence rate of 1 in 9000 live births in the U.S., the authors suggest that an association with fetal exposure to alcohol be seriously considered. This association is strengthened by a second case of EBA reported in an FAS infant who also showed renal abnormalities (Dunigan and Werlin, 1981). Corrective surgery did not improve the bile flow and the infant died.

IMMUNOLOGIC

Children with FAS have increased susceptibility to life-threatening bacterial infections, as well as to minor infectious diseases. Structural abnormalities, including small bones in the base of the skull, may cause morphologic problems of the nasal sinuses which predispose them to obstruction and infection. Johnson (1979) examined an FAS infant who presented at 4 months with a persistent, severely stuffed nose and otitis media. Despite vigorous treatment with antibiotics and decongestants, the symptoms persisted. Skull X-rays revealed hypoplastic sphenoid and ethnoid sinuses with small posterior nasal canals.

Infections were evaluated in 13 FAS children, aged 12 months to 10½ years, who were matched by age and sex to a control group of normal children and an additional group of SGA patients (Johnson et al, 1981). More infectious disease occurred among the FAS cases, and the majority had repeated episodes of otitis media and upper respiratory infections. Two had bacterial meningitis; five others required hospitalization for lobar consolidated pneumonia and three for gastroenteritis. Immune deficiencies were common. Absolute lymphocyte counts were depressed for both alcohol and SGA groups, suggesting that intrauterine growth is associated with lymphopenia. Mitogen-induced synthesis of T-cells was depressed in the alcohol group but not in the SGA children. Similarly, abnormal quantitative immunoglobulin levels were observed in 9 of the FAS cases and none of the controls. The authors suggest that intrauterine exposure to ethanol is teratogenic to the immune system. The effects did not appear to be related to the degree of growth retardation or malnutrition and did not seem to correct with age. Similar effects were observed on the immune system of the rat; however the effects were transient and not evident at 18 months (Monjan and Mandell, 1980).

CUTANEOUS

Modifications in dermatoglyphics occur in the ulnar and radial loops and whorls in the fingertips, the palmar creases, and the hallucal area (Qazi et al, 1980; Tanaka et al, 1981). Changes in digital and palmar creases result from flexional folding of the palmar skin and occur in the second and third gestational month. Alterations in dermal ridges reflect growth disturbances during the third and fourth months of gestation.

Early case reports cited hemangiomas and hirsutism in infancy

(Clarren and Smith, 1978). Hair whorls have been observed to tend toward counterclockwise rather than clockwise rotation (Dehaene, personal communication). Relationships between the development of hair patterns and the central nervous system have been reported (Smith and Gong, 1974). The most critical gestational period for scalp hair pattern development is 10–12 weeks.

TUMORS

Several neoplasms have been reported in association with FAS. Adrenal carcinoma was reported in one 12-year-old FAS patient (Hornstein et al, 1977). A clinically unsuspected paravertebral neuroblastoma was discovered on autopsy of a 110-day-old male severely affected with FAS who died of aspiration with early pneumonia (Kinney et al, 1980). Another sympathoblastoma was observed in a six-day-old FAS male (Ponte et al, 1982). An embryonal rhabdomyosarcoma of the urinary bladder was found in a 21-month-old male (Becker et al, 1982). Liver cancer was diagnosed in a 27-month-old male, 20 months after a renal transplant (Khan et al, 1979). Ganglioneuroblastomas were observed in two children with fetal hydantoin and fetal alcohol syndromes (Ramilo and Harris, 1979; Seeler et al, 1979).

The presence of carcinomas in FAS patients is rare, and there is no uniformity in the nature of the tumors which have been reported. Fetal hydantoin syndrome has been associated with an increased frequency of neuroblastoma. FAS and fetal hydantoin syndrome demonstrate many similar characteristics, which suggests common mechanisms. Although conclusions cannot be drawn about causality, embryonic tumors are uncommon occurrences and alcohol's role in their etiology should not be overlooked.

Clinical studies

Multiple anomalies have been reported in case studies of FAS. In some prospective studies, a higher incidence of birth defects has been observed in the infants of heavy drinkers, but no pattern has emerged. Among 163 infants, Hanson et al (1978) observed signs compatible with prenatal effects of alcohol on growth and morphology in 9 neonates whose mothers had consumed more than 1 oz AA per day. Two of these babies were born to alcoholics and were diagnosed as FAS. Two additional babies born to nondrinkers showed signs of FAE. Infants were examined in pairs, selected for maternal drinking pattern, delivery date, and hospital of birth. Infants were rated abnormal if they had either small palpebral fissures or multiple dysmorphic features in conjunction with microcephaly or SGA. The individual abnormalities were not described.

Studies in Cleveland and Boston also observed an increased incidence of congenital anomalies among infants of alcohol abusers. Sokol et al (1980) reported that 16 of 42 infants born to alcohol abusers had at least one major or minor anomaly. Abnormalities were observed in genitourinary, cutaneous, cardiac, oral, and skeletal systems. At Boston City Hospital, in the first cohort, major or minor anomalies were observed in 29 of 42 neonates born to heavy drinkers (Ouellette et al, 1977). Multiple anomalies occurred more frequently in children of heavy drinkers. In another cohort, one major or three minor anomalies were found in 3 infants of 25 heavy drinkers (Rosett et al, 1983b). While more neonates of heavy drinkers exhibited abnormalities, no specific pattern was noted in either cohort. Because of the small number of babies exhibiting abnormalities, an analysis of the effects of other confounding variables was not possible. In contrast, three studies by Kaminski et al (1981) did not demonstrate any relationships between alcohol use and major congenital malformations. The discrepancy may have resulted from the small number of heavy drinkers and the relative infrequency and multiplicity of abnormalities.

Experimental research

Most of the fetal anomalies clinically observed in association with maternal alcohol abuse have been produced in experimental animals: mice, miniature swine, dogs, and sheep have developed facial, cardiac, renal, genitourinary, and skeletal abnormalities (Chernoff, 1977; Randall et al, 1977b; Randall and Taylor, 1979; Ellis and Pick, 1980; Dexter et al, 1980; Potter et al, 1980). Experiments have been conducted to answer several questions: Are effects dependent on dose? Are they related to gestational stage of exposure? Is there variance with genetic strain? Does alcohol have direct effects or is maldevelopment secondary to malnutrition or illnesses? What is the role of acetaldehyde?

DOSE RESPONSE

Chernoff (1977) developed a mouse model to simulate chronic maternal alcoholism. Offspring of mothers exposed to alcohol throughout pregnancy demonstrated a pattern of abnormalities similar to FAS. Low birthweight, deficient occiput ossification, neural anomalies, cardiac defects, and eyelid dysmorphology occurred with a dose-response effect. Teratogenic dose levels differed among strains of mice. Fetal blood alcohol levels were similar to maternal levels but varied among species following exposure to equivalent doses (Chernoff, 1980). CBA mice demonstrated less ADH activity, higher blood alcohol levels, and more malformations than C3H or C57 mice.

Malformations in beagle dogs differed in nature and severity when alcohol was increased from 2.1 g/kg per day to 12 g/kg per day (Ellis and Pick, 1980). Experimental bitches ($N = 28$) received ethanol by gastric intubation and had free access to a standard dry diet. Controls ($N = 10$) were given equi-caloric doses of sucrose by gastric intubation and were pair fed. Pups born to bitches exposed to 2.1 g/kg per day twice daily on days 14–30 demonstrated morphologic abnormalities, including cleft palate, absent kidney, kink tail, and opening of the urethra into the abdominal cavity. Offspring of controls had no abnormalities. Higher doses were associated with spontaneous abortions, increasing amounts of growth retardation, and morphologic anomalies as well as early mortality.

Rasmussen and Christensen (1980) observed a clear dose-effect relationship in frequency of malformation in the mouse, but no morphologic difference in the nature of the defects. Randall et al (1981) compared the effects of three doses of alcohol in the mouse fetus. The rate of malformations increased as the dose increased from 20% to 25% and to 30%. Mortality and resorptions were highest in the group exposed to 30%. Experiments which have employed low doses of alcohol have demonstrated no teratogenic effects in mice, rats, or rabbits (Øisund et al, 1978; Samson et al, 1979; Schwetz et al, 1978). In chicken embryos, high ethanol doses were lethal, whereas lesser doses were neither toxic nor teratogenic (Koda et al, 1980).

Response to alcohol may depend upon the route and regimen of administration as well as the dose (Lochry et al, 1982). In experimental models, alcohol has been administered intraperitoneally, intravenously, by intubation, in an all liquid diet, or as the liquid in a lab chow diet. Maximum blood alcohol levels and the duration of exposure vary according to the technique. Peak BACs of 227 mg percent occurred in C3H mice following oral administration of 5 g/kg, with levels falling close to zero within a few hours. At this level, sedative effects were observed. When 5.8 g/kg were administered by intraperitoneal injections, C57 mice were rendered comatose with BACs reaching 800 mg percent. Anomalies have been observed only when the dose was sufficient to cause a blood alcohol level of at least 150 mg percent, which exceeds the legal level of intoxication in humans (Abel and Greizerstein, 1982).

GESTATIONAL STAGE

Most studies seek to replicate daily drinking with consistent exposure to high doses of alcohol, but some have modeled binge drinking by administering ethanol on specific gestational days. Eyes and limbs were affected when fetal mice were exposed to alcohol on days 8–10 (Kronick, 1976). Fetal mortality increased following treatment on days 9–12. Similarly, limb abnormalities occurred following exposure of mice to alcohol on days 9–11 (Webster et al, 1980). Exposure on day 7 and 8 caused exencephaly and maxillary hypoplasia. Sulik et al (1981) administered 5.8 g/kg in two doses 4 hours apart on day 7. Facial anomalies similar to FAS were observed in the mouse fetus seven days after exposure.

When a single dose of 5 g/kg was administered to the mouse through intragastric intubation, growth was retarded but neither the nature nor the severity of soft tissue anomalies was affected (Lochry et al, 1982). Skeletal and cardiac defects were not evaluated. A single moderate dose of ethanol (0.02 ml/g body weight) administered peritoneally on either day 6, 9, or 12 did not significantly affect embryonic development in the rat (Varma and Persaud, 1979).

The incidence and nature of malformations depends on gestational stage at the time of exposure as well as on blood alcohol levels. Webster et al (1983) observed malformations in C57 mice when blood alcohol levels were 400 mg percent or more. Alcohol in equivalent doses was administered by intraperitoneal injections or by intubation. Lower peak BACs followed oral administration and caused fewer anomalies. The nature of the malformations depended on the day of treatment, while severity and frequency depended on BACs. Facial abnormalities followed treatment on days 7 and 8; limb defects were associated with exposure on days 9 and 10.

GENETIC SUSCEPTIBILITY

Strain differences in susceptibility suggest a genetic component to toxicity. Chernoff (1980) observed that both maternal blood alcohol levels and the incidence of abnormalities were related to the strain of mouse. Among three strains, CBA mice were most severely affected, C3H next, and C57 least affected by exposure to a diet in which 20% of the calories were ethanol. The incidence of abnormalities was inversely related to maternal alcohol dehydrogenase activity and directly associated with microsomal ethanol oxidizing system (MEOS). Giknis et al (1980) also reported that the teratogenicity of ethanol was dose dependent, although somewhat modified by genetic determinants in four mouse strains.

Differences may be related either to genetically determined enzyme levels which influence BAC and acetaldehyde metabolism or to inborn tissue sensitivities to teratogenic agents. The genetic predisposition to dysmorphology following exposure to high concentrations of alcohol differs greatly between species and even between inbred strains of mice. Riley and Lochry (1982) observed that CBA mice were more affected than C3H mice even when BACs were substantially lower. Sulik et al (1981) noted that C57 mice have a genetic predisposition for the facial anomalies induced by alcohol: 12% of the control animals demonstrated ocular defects. Rats demonstrate growth and behavioral changes, but few morphologic abnormalities.

In humans there is no evidence of race-related susceptibility to the teratogenic effects of alcohol. Fetal alcohol syndrome occurs in every ethnic group. The incidence of FAS is related to the chronicity and severity of maternal alcoholism, and it increases with the rate of alcohol abuse within the population. Drinking patterns within ethnic groups undoubtedly are determined by cultural as well as genetic factors. Individual differences in fetal susceptibility as well as in maternal metabolism of alcohol affect outcome. Evidence for variation in fetal susceptibility in humans is found in sets of fraternal twins in which one infant is more affected than the other (Christoffel and Salafsky, 1975; Santolaya et al, 1978).

DIRECT EFFECTS OF ALCOHOL

The direct effects of alcohol have been demonstrated in in vitro studies in which rat embryos growing in a tissue culture medium were exposed on days 9½ to 11½ to either 0.15 or 0.3 grams percent of alcohol (Brown et al, 1979). Dose-dependent retardation in growth and differentiation occurred as a direct effect of alcohol in the absence of altered maternal nutrition, metabolism, or physiology. Structural deficiencies were attributed to a reduced number of cells. Impaired cellular proliferation has been suggested as the mechanism of action of other teratogenic agents, such as those that cause cleft palate (Scott, 1977).

Alcohol has direct effects on the molecular structure of the phospholipid bilayers of cell membranes, and it increases cell membrane fluidity (Chin et al, 1979). Ethanol's effects were concentration-related in BACs ranging from 1–16 mg/ml (in humans 1 mg/ml is equivalent to the legal level of intoxication). Although this fluidizing effect is small, the disturbance in normal lipo-protein structure could alter cell proliferation, migration, and physiology.

EFFECTS OF ACETALDEHYDE

Acetaldehyde, which may be 1000 times more embryotoxic than ethanol, also plays a critical role in teratogenesis. Intravenous injections of acetaldehyde doses of 0.05 or 0.10 ml on gestational days 7, 8, and 9 caused resorptions, growth retardation, and CNS and cardiovascular abnormalities in mouse embryos on day 10 (O'Shea and Kaufman, 1979). The most common defect was failure of the cranial and caudal regions of the neural tube to close. Further study demonstrated that treatment on several successive days was more embryotoxic and teratogenic than was a single exposure (O'Shea and Kaufman, 1981). The extent of the abnormalities was dose dependent. On day 19, growth retardation persisted, but no congenital anomalies were observed in the surviving fetuses. Similarly, a high resorption rate followed injection of maternal mice with acetaldehyde (Dreosti et al, 1981). Surviving fetuses were normal but weighed substantially less than controls. In both studies, resorption sites were adjacent to healthy fetuses, suggesting selective sensitivity to acetaldehyde.

Intraperitoneal administration of acetaldehyde to pregnant CF rats on gestational days 10, 11, and 12 resulted in multiple fetal abnormalities on day 21 (Sreenathan et al, 1982). Single and triple doses of 50, 75, and 100 mg/kg were injected. Fetal and placental growth retardation, facial and limb anomalies, and mortality occurred more often following exposure to continued doses than to a single dose. There was marked variability of effect within litters, suggesting individual variability in susceptibility to acetaldehyde free of ethanol.

Acetaldehyde has been difficult to study in vivo because of difficulties measuring its concentration in blood. New biochemical techniques should help to clarify its significance (Lindros, 1983). Since acetaldehyde is oxidized very rapidly in the presence of aldehyde dehydrogenase, in some studies that enzyme has been inhibited by adding disulfiram. When disulfiram and alcohol were administered separately and in combination to fetal rats on days 7 and 16, neither agent by itself had a significant effect on fetal growth and development (Véghelyi et al, 1978). The combined action of disulfiram and alcohol caused increased fetal resorption and skeletal retardation and decreased fetal weight. No effects were observed when the concentrations of acetaldehyde were below 35 μM—the peak level which normally occurs following moderate alcohol use. Webster et al (1983) also did not observe abnormalities in mice embryos following acute exposure to doses of acetaldehyde lower than those which occur with alcohol abuse.

In vitro exposure of 9.5 day rat embryos to acetaldehyde (4.5 μM–45 μM) induced malformations similar to those seen in association with exposure to alcohol (Popov et al, 1981). Exposure of 10 day rat embryos to acetaldehyde in vitro caused retarded growth and development with a concentration response (Campbell and Fantel, 1983). No effects were observed at 5 μM; embryotoxicity began with doses of 25 μM; lethality was evident at 100 μM. Embryos exposed to 25, 50, or 75 μM acetaldehyde contained significantly less protein and decreased DNA. Head growth was specifically compromised.

The effects of acetaldehyde have only been observed with high blood concentrations. In humans, this occurs with consumption of large volumes of alcohol, particularly in chronic alcoholics with hepatic damage.

INDIRECT EFFECTS OF ALCOHOL

Alcohol and/or acetaldehyde may indirectly induce growth retardation and morphologic abnormalities by altering the maternal-placental system. Majewski (1981) observed that the stage of alcoholism is a more important determinant of fetal outcome than is the amount of absolute alcohol consumed. Véghelyi et al (1978) noted that many mothers of FAS children had liver disease during pregnancy. Most were older mothers, between 31 and 34 years when the affected child was born. Rarely was the FAS child their first born. Dehaene et al (1981) observed that FAS occurs in children of multiparous women suffering from chronic, complicated alcoholism. May and Hymbaugh (1982) noted that the rate of mortality (21%) was higher among FAS mothers than among other women. Clarren (1982) reported that 75% of the natural mothers were missing or dead within 5 years of giving birth to an FAS child.

Individual women repeatedly bear FAS or FAE children (May and Hymbaugh, 1982). Fitze et al (1978) reported that retardation was increasingly severe in each of four successive children born to an alcoholic woman. The extent of fetal damage was also observed to increase with parity in several other families (Manzke and Grosse, 1975; Iosub et al, 1981; Bierich et al, 1976; Palmer et al, 1974). Dexter et al (1983) observed progressive severity of alcohol's effects in three serial litters of miniature swine. Growth retardation and stillbirths increased with the duration of chronic consumption of alcohol (> 3 g/kg/day), even in the presence of adequate nutrition.

Experimental studies have attempted to separate the direct effects of alcohol from secondary effects of undernutrition. A careful pair-feeding study in mice has shown that restricted caloric intake, by itself, was not teratogenic (Randall et al, 1981). However, dietary intake is only one determinant of nutritional state. Some of alcohol's effects on morphology may result from impaired absorption and cellular utilization of essential nutrients.

Alcohol's interference with the active transport of amino acids across the rat placenta may result in selective malnutrition of the fetus despite adequate maternal dietary intake (Fisher et al, 1981; Henderson et al, 1981; Lin, 1981). Fisher et al (1982) demonstrated inhibitory effects on amino acid uptake only at very high concentrations of alcohol and acetaldehyde in examinations of healthy term human placental slices. Similar dose-response effects had not been reported in rodent experiments. Since there are structural differences between primate and rodent placentas, experiments in monkeys are needed to clarify dose-response effects.

In addition to its effects on placental transfer of proteins, ethanol inhibits the synthesis of fetal protein. Changes in ornithine decarboxylase (ODC) activity in the heart and brain of fetal and neonatal rats exposed to alcohol from gestational day 11 on have been observed (Thadani et al, 1977). These enzymatic changes alter polyamine metabolism involved in protein formation. Cardiac protein synthesis has also been shown to be inhibited in fetal rat hearts (Rawat, 1979). Henderson et al (1980) demonstrated that placental 14 c-valine uptake was reduced in the rat following both chronic and acute alcohol exposure. Fetal rats exposed to alcohol throughout gestation had decreased body and organ weights as well as increased postnatal mortality. RNA levels in brain, heart, kidney, and liver were decreased. Net protein synthesis was reduced in both maternal and fetal tissues when blood ethanol levels were higher than 3.2 mg/ml. Ethanol-induced hypothermia was a major contributor to this phenomenon. In the presence of hypothermia, BACs of 0.83 mg/ml caused a reduction in net protein synthesis. Dreosti et al (1981) observed that incorporation of 3H-thymidine into DNA in brain and liver tissue was reduced following exposure to high levels of ethanol or to moderate concentrations of acetaldehyde (1–2 mg/100 ml).

Teratogenic effects of ethanol may be heightened by the nutritional deficiencies associated with chronic alcoholism. Deficiencies of zinc and other minerals and vitamins have been experimentally demonstrated to result in retarded fetal growth, congenital malformations, and increased fetal resorption and mortality (McClain and Su, 1983). Calcium, magnesium, and zinc, as well as folate, may be depleted as a consequence of increased urinary excretion, loss due to vomiting and diarrhea, and inadequate intake (Flink, 1971). A 100% increase in urinary excretion of calcium and a 167% increase in magnesium excretion have been observed to begin within 20 minutes of ingestion of 30 ml of ethanol by normal volunteers and to continue for about 2 hours. Magnesium has important roles in fetal development since it stabilizes DNA and RNA, binds sRNA to the ribosome, and is involved in the activating and transfer systems of all amino acids.

Zinc is required for RNA and DNA synthesis and for a number of metallo-enzymes, including carbonic anhydrase and alcohol dehydrogenase. Prenatal zinc deficiencies in the rat were associated with growth retardation and congenital malformations similar to that seen with FAS (Hurley, 1979). Zinc-deficient diets were teratogenic when administered on days 0–10, 6–14, or throughout gestation. Maternal plasma zinc levels fell rapidly when diets were zinc-deficient but quickly returned to original values after zinc was refed. Concentrations of zinc in postpartum maternal plasma and milk were normal. The short period of zinc deficiency caused a high rate of stillbirths and neonatal mortality, and a high incidence of congenital anomalies and low birthweight.

Acute and long-term exposure to ethanol reduced placental and fetal uptake of zinc in rats (Ghishan et al, 1982). In animals treated with ethanol chronically (gestational days 4–20), decreased total fetal body concentrations of zinc led to decreased fetal protein synthesis and reduced growth. Lowered plasma zinc levels in alcoholic pregnant women were associated with fetal dysmorphogenesis (Flynn et al, 1981). While maternal and fetal-cord-plasma zinc levels were both lower, abnormalities were correlated only with maternal-plasma zinc levels. Low maternal-plasma zinc levels have been reported in association with abnormalities and growth retardation by others (Meadows et al, 1981; Cavdar, 1983).

The role of zinc has not been consistently confirmed. Henderson et al (1979) reported that decreased body, brain, heart, kidney, and liver weights observed in Sprague-Dawley rats were not due to zinc deficiency. Chronic exposure to ethanol in doses sufficient to produce intoxication had no effect on maternal bone and brain zinc levels or on fetal bone and muscle zinc concentrations at 20 days' gestation. Jones et al (1981) found no differences between alcohol exposed rats and pair-fed or ad libitum controls in fetal uptake of zinc or of the analogs of glucose and amino acid. Growth retardation was observed but was not considered to be due to impaired transfer of nutrients. The differences in the findings may reflect dose and regimen of administration, stages of fetal development, nutritional considerations, or difficulties in measuring zinc concentrations. Transient periods of zinc deprivation which can disrupt fetal development cannot be identified without sequential measurements.

The teratogenic effects of ethanol may be exacerbated by dietary deficiencies. Ruth and Goldsmith (1981) observed anomalies in rat pups whose zinc-deprived mothers were treated with a single intraperitoneal dose of ethanol. Neither the ethanol alone nor the deprivation of zinc caused these abnormalities.

Tanaka et al (1982c) have suggested that administering zinc with ethanol prevents the damage that would be caused by ethanol alone. Pups born to Wistar rats who received 30% of their calories as ethanol with zinc from gestational days 0–19 demonstrated less growth retardation, lower resorption rates, and higher protein content in the cerebrum than rats fed ethanol alone. Administration of zinc resulted in higher maternal zinc levels but no increase in fetal cerebral zinc. Administration of 5% glucose late in gestation to the ethanol-fed rats resulted in higher fetal cerebral weights. Although fetal development was less disturbed when alcohol was administered with zinc or glucose, it did not reach the level of the controls.

Ethanol also causes impaired intestinal absorption of folic acid. Sullivan and Herbert (1964) demonstrated that hematologic response to folic acid therapy was repeatedly prevented by the concomitant administration of whiskey, wine, or laboratory ethanol. When body stores are decreased and dietary intake is poor, ethanol may act as a weak folate antagonist. Folate antagonists have been shown to cause fetal resorption, stillbirths, and congenital malformations in the rat (Sullivan, 1967). Folic acid and magnesium have produced a variety of skeletal and soft tissue anomalies in the rat (Hurley, 1979). Human fetal malformations have also been associated with a dietary deficiency of folate (Lindenbaum, 1974).

Alcohol-induced alterations in fetal endocrine function may affect fetal development through changes in levels of placental tropic hormones, prolactin and oxytocin, adrenal cortical hormones, maternal and fetal thyroid and sex hormones, and maternal insulin (Anderson, 1981). While few studies have examined the effects of alcohol ingestion on maternal endocrine balance during pregnancy, ethanol's known adverse effects on the menstrual cycle and fertility suggest effects during gestation. Alcohol has been observed to be a gonadal toxin in the rat (Van Thiel et al, 1977). Alcohol exposure beginning on gestational day 100 depressed pituitary thyroid function and increased adrenal cortical function in fetal ewes (Rose et al, 1981). Crown–rump lengths and body weights were lowered, suggesting that growth is inhibited by chronic exposure in the third trimester.

Effects of alcohol on placental production and synthesis of hormones in the human remain unclear. Sheean (1983) found no alcohol effects on placental endocrine metabolism. The enzymatic function of microsomes extracted from placentae of seven heavy drinkers, seven light drinkers, and seven controls were compared. There were no significant differences in the kinetics of the placental aromatase complex, which is active in the formation of steroid hormones and maintenance of pregnancy. The author concluded that reduction in placental estrogen formation is not responsible for growth retardation. More study is needed since the period of abstinence preceding labor and delivery might have been ample time for the recovery of the enzymatic functions. In the mouse only 24 hours is needed for recovery of hepatic microsomal cytochrome P-450 concentrations after acute experimental exposure to ethanol (Pennington et al, 1978).

RESTITUTION

Compensatory development and restitution can occur in rodents when acute exposure to alcohol ceases. During the early stages of organogenesis, there is a capacity for recovery from severe damage and from developmental retardation (Snow and Tam, 1979). Much of the recovery occurs within 48 hours of the inflicted damage. It is accomplished by a period of accelerated development during which the embryo may be particularly vulnerable to stress. The abnormal embryogenesis apparent on day 9 in rats exposed to high doses of alcohol on gestational days 5–8 was not apparent on day 20 (Anders and Persaud, 1980). Similar observations were made in rats exposed to acetaldehyde (O'Shea and Kaufman, 1981; Dreosti, 1981). The incidence of defects was much lower when examination was on the twelfth day rather than on the tenth, with no difference in resorption rates. This suggests that the blastocyst is capable of considerable compensatory growth and repair before development is completed.

Summary

Multiple mechanisms underlie alcohol's effects in utero. The teratogenic effects of ethanol may be viewed as an extension of the pathophysiologic manifestations of chronic alcoholism. Biochemical and pharmacologic effects of ethanol and its metabolites disturb fetal development directly and alter the maternal-placental-fetal system. Rapidly growing and organizing tissues show the effects with little delay. The complete FAS probably represents the cumulative result of multiple adverse effects throughout gestation. Variability in the nature and severity of effects is determined by differences in tissue sensitivity, duration of exposure, stage of gestation, dose levels, and ability to metabolize ethanol. Exposure at crucial developmental stages will affect the structure and form of particular systems. During the first trimester, alcohol may alter cell membranes and the embryonic organization of tissues. Throughout gestation, alcohol's effects on the metabolism of proteins, lipids, and carbohydrates can retard cell growth and division. Alcohol also interferes with active transport of amino acids across the placenta, reducing the availability of essential nutrients to the fetus. Particular organ systems may be most vulnerable at the time of their most rapid cell division. Susceptibility may be related to small differences in the genetic capacity to metabolize alcohol and in tissue sensitivity. However, it is the consumption of large amounts of alcohol and high BACs that are critical. In no instance, in either clinical or experimental reports, have persistent effects of consumption of low levels of alcohol been observed.

Six

Brain and Behavior

The developing central nervous system is vulnerable throughout gestation to the effects of high concentrations of alcohol. Abnormalities of the CNS are particularly critical since they disrupt intellectual and behavioral development. The most severe FAS patients demonstrate profound and persistent mental retardation and behavioral disturbances. Sleep disturbances, delays in mental and motor development, hyperactivity, language dysfunction, and altered evoked potentials on the electroencephalogram (EEG) have been reported in the children of women who drank heavily during pregnancy. Some of these nonspecific symptoms have been observed in the absence of facial dysmorphology and growth retardation. Alcohol's effects on behavior, brain structure, electrical activity, neurochemistry, and neuroendocrine regulation have been studied in offspring of chronic alcoholic mothers and in experimental animals.

Intelligence

In 1968, Lemoine et al reported intellectual impairment and psychomotor hyperactivity with developmental delay among 127 children of chronic alcoholic parents. Their average IQ was approximately 70; average age for standing was one year and for walking was 20 months. While initial syllables were uttered at normal dates, first words were pronounced poorly and phrases were slow in coming.

The children were quarrelsome and irritable as they grew older. During school years, learning delays were common.

Reports from other case series confirm observations of mental retardation among offspring of chronic alcoholics. A retrospective review of the charts of the Perinatal Project of the National Institute of Neurologic Disease and Stroke revealed lower IQs among children of alcohol dependent women (Jones et al, 1974). The project investigated 55,000 pregnancies with a seven year followup of offspring at 12 medical centers. Direct questions about alcohol use had not been asked but mention of alcohol abuse appeared in prenatal records of 69 women. In 23, there was evidence of chronic alcoholism before and during pregnancy. Reduced weight, length, and head circumference were observed in the newborn nursery and at age 7 among the children exposed to alcohol in utero. IQ testing at age 7 was available for 12 children of alcoholic women: six who had lived with their mothers had a mean IQ of 73, and six who had spent some time with relatives had a mean IQ of 84.

Retardation was also prevalent among 52 children with FAS whose cases were retrospectively reviewed in Sweden: 58% had IQs below 85 and 19% below 70 (Kyllerman et al, 1979; Olegård et al, 1979). An extended study of 21 of the youngest children demonstrated a nonspecific discoordinated motor pattern with a lack of precision and plasticity. In addition, cerebral palsy occurred in 8.3% of the children, compared with 0.2% in the population as a whole.

Shurygin (1974) evaluated 42 children of 18 alcoholic mothers and found disturbances in the developing CNS of those whose mothers drank during pregnancy. Among 23 children (aged 9 months to 20 years) born after their mothers had developed full-fledged alcoholism, 14 were mentally retarded and many demonstrated signs of organic impairment of the CNS early in infancy. In contrast, 19 children (aged 12–32), born before their mothers had developed full-fledged alcoholism, demonstrated emotional and behavioral disorders which developed around age 9 or 10 and tended to remit after their social environment was improved.

In a series of 20 FAS patients ranging in age from 9 months to 21 years, Streissguth et al (1978a) found that retardation was greatest in the patients with the most severe facial dysmorphology. The mean IQ was 65, with a range from 16 to 105. The IQ of 60% of the group was more than 2 SD below the mean. Evaluation one to four years later revealed that the mean IQ remained relatively stable over time (Streissguth et al, 1978b).

Others have also observed that the lowest IQs and the poorest prognoses occur in the most severely dysmorphic children. Dehaene et al (1977b) reported that the average IQ of 22 FAS children was 66, with a range from 33 to 112. The most severely dysmorphic scored in the range of 60 and did not improve over time. Initially low scores for five children with less severe dysmorphism reached the more or less normal range of 80 to 90. Majewski (1981) observed similar scores among 18 FAS patients ranging in age from 3.5 to 9 years. The average IQ in the five with the most severe dysmorphology (AEIII) was 66 (range 50–95); in four moderate cases (AEII) the mean was 79 (range 47–102); and among 9 diagnosed as mild (AEI) the mean was 91 (range 61–130).

Bayley Scales of Mental and Motor Development were administered to 462 infants at 8 months of age to evaluate the effects of maternal alcohol, nicotine, and caffeine use during pregnancy (Streissguth et al, 1980). Moderate alcohol use was reported to be associated with decreased mental and motor development in multiple regression analysis adjusted for effects of nicotine, caffeine, gestational age, parity, and maternal education. All of the variables measured in the multiple regression analysis accounted for 5–6% of the total variance in the Bayley Scale scores: alcohol use accounted for 1–2%. The table of mental and motor scores presented by the authors grouped women in drinking categories which were not mutually exclusive; women ingesting very different amounts of alcohol were all considered as one group. The mental scores of ten infants born to mothers who reported drinking more than 4 oz AA a day were included four times in categories from 1 oz or more to 4 oz or more. When developmental measures are analyzed by specific dose and each infant is included only once, the mean mental scores of the infants born to mothers drinking the most (4 oz AA or more per day) is 98 (normal range). The mean mental score for all other drinking categories is 116 (1 SD above the mean) (see Table 6-1). Among the ten women who consumed more than 4 oz AA daily, one reported drinking 25 oz a day, and eight were consuming more than 10 drinks a day. Thus, our interpretation of these findings is that the decrement in IQ occurred only in the children of women who were drinking very heavily. At eight months, there was no measurable effect in the offspring of women who were drinking less than 4 oz AA a day.

Bayley Scales of Mental and Motor Development were significantly lower (20 points) at one year among 12 infants born to

Table 6-1 Mental scores at 8 months and maternal alcohol use
in month prior to pregnancy

MEAN DAILY ABSOLUTE ALCOHOL SCORE (OZ AA)		N	MEAN MENTAL SCORES
		MATERNAL DRINKING: OVERLAPPING CATEGORIES	
≤0.1		216	116
<1.0 (0.0–1.0)		365	116
≥1.0 (1.0–25.0)		97	114
≥2.0 (2.0–25.0)		25	109
≥3.0 (3.0–25.0)		12	101
≥4.0 (4.0–25.0)		10	98
	Total:	462	116
		MATERNAL DRINKING: MUTUALLY EXCLUSIVE CATEGORIES	
≤0.1		216	116
0.1–0.99		149	116
1.0–1.9		72	116
2.0–2.9		13	116
3.0–3.9		2	116
4.0–25.0		10	98
	Total:	462	116

Adapted from Streissguth et al, 1980.

women who had been diagnosed during pregnancy as alcohol abusers (Golden et al, 1982). All had been identified at birth as FAS or
possible FAS cases. Compared to non-alcohol abusing controls
matched for gestational age, sex, and race, the alcohol-exposed
group demonstrated an excess frequency of abnormalities, growth
retardation, and microcephaly at birth and at one year of age. These
findings suggest that the children at risk for developmental delays
are the severely affected infants who demonstrate physical abnormalities.

Activity and learning

The earliest and largest prospective evaluation of the effects of maternal alcohol consumption on behavior and development was un-

dertaken in Seattle (Streissguth et al, 1981). This large body of work represents most of the prospective research that has been undertaken on the effects of alcohol on intellectual capacity. Careful observations were made on children at several stages of life, beginning with the neonate. A followup cohort of 250 heavier drinkers and smokers and 250 infrequent drinkers and abstainers were selected from 1529 women who had been interviewed during pregnancy.

In order to minimize the impact of differences in environment and mother–infant interactions, initial testing was done in the hospital during the first two days of life. The Neonatal Behavior Assessment Scale (Brazelton, 1973) was administered to 417 infants, 92% of whom were between 9 and 35 hours old (mean age, 27 hours) (Streissguth et al, 1983a). Maternal alcohol use in mid-pregnancy was related to decreased habituation and "low arousal" after adjustment for seven confounding variables. The magnitude of the effects was dose related, with infants of women who drank more than 2 oz AA per day most severely affected. The significance of differences at this age is questionable since the Brazelton examination is standardized for the third day of life but not earlier.

Naturalistic observations of 124 infants from the Seattle cohort identified subtle differences between children of heavy drinkers and controls (Landesman-Dwyer et al, 1978). Increased maternal alcohol use was significantly related to the following infant behaviors ($p < 0.05$): increased head turnings to the left, tremulousness, hand to face movement, time with eyes opened, and decreased vigorous body activity. These associations were independent of nicotine, sex, and birthweight.

Operant head turning and sucking at two days were studied in two different subsets of infants ($N = 225$, $N = 80$). In multiple regression analyses, there were no significant alcohol main effects but there were significant alcohol by nicotine interactions for head turning tasks (Martin et al, 1977). The combination of maternal drinking and smoking resulted in poorer infant learning than did either variable alone. Heavier alcohol use was also related to decreased sucking pressure in 151 neonates (Martin et al, 1979).

The relationships between these findings and future development are not clear. Different subsets of the original cohort were examined in each behavioral study due to logistical problems. It is not clear whether the same children exhibited abnormalities in each study since no data has been published on the relationship between the

performances of individual infants on different tests. Performance
during the first 2 days of life is not compared with performance
studied at 8 months and at 4 years. There is no indication whether
developmental catch-up occurs, or if early differences portend later
problems. Recent animal experiments suggest that some differences
in the alcohol-exposed offspring represent a delay in development
which reverses with maturity (see experimental section below). Researchers conducting pilot studies must look for extremely subtle
alterations in behavior while also acknowledging that they may be
transient and of little clinical significance. Followup studies of these
specific children are required to determine the meaning of effects
observed in infancy.

Landesman-Dwyer et al (1981) examined long term behavioral
correlates of moderate social drinking and cigarette use during pregnancy in 128 children at 4 years of age. This was a subset of a group
of 801 middle-class women whose alcohol consumption and smoking had been studied during pregnancy (Little, 1977). Average alcohol consumption of the moderate social drinkers was 0.88 oz AA
per day prior to pregnancy and 0.45 oz AA per day during the fourth
month of pregnancy. Women who drank more than 2.5 oz AA per
day were eliminated from the study. Significant associations occurred between the mother's drinking during pregnancy and the
child's attention and social compliance at four years. These differences were independent of factors in the home measured by a standardized test. However, maternal use of alcohol and cigarettes during the four years after birth was not investigated. No assessment of
maternal personality or of the child's medical history was made.
Further investigation is needed to determine whether differences in
the observed child behaviors were due to prenatal or postnatal factors. It is also unclear whether the slight differences detected in the
children's attention, social compliance, and fidgetiness will persist
or will affect later performance.

Of 87 children attending a Learning Disorders Unit in New
Haven, 15 were found to have mothers with a history of alcoholism
during pregnancy (Shaywitz et al, 1980). The children were born
to ten mothers, of whom two had died and four were hospitalized
for disorders related to alcoholism. At the time of testing, the children ranged in age from 6½ to 18½ years. The children's growth was
retarded and they had mild facial dysmorphology. Their average
IQ was 98, with a range of 82 to 113. Despite the normal range of

IQs, there were persistent learning problems characterized by attentional deficits and hyperactivity. Differences in cognitive performance between these 15 children and the 72 other children attending the Learning Disorders Unit were not discussed. The older children demonstrated less severe dysmorphic features and higher IQs, which suggested to the authors that these were milder cases. An alternative hypothesis would be amelioration of the effects.

Bierich (1978) observed restlessness and an inability to concentrate, as well as a lack of initiative in FAS children. Their learning ability and other mental functions improved when their hyperexcitability subsided. Patient, long-term occupational therapy was beneficial to children who had not suffered severe damage. Koranyi and Csiky (1978) reported 5 cases of FAS ranging in age from 21 months to 13 years. Medical and educational intervention alleviated physical and mental retardation but normal levels were not attained. They concluded that mental symptomatology can be altered by socioeconomic conditions, maternal–infant interactions, state of health, and the timeliness of intervention.

Steinhausen et al (1982) reported mean IQ (89) and social maturity (71) scores among 32 FAS cases (aged 4–10 years), identified during a three year period in Berlin, that were significantly lower than in 28 healthy controls. Visual perception and psycholinguistic development were also impaired. Birthweight and intelligence correlated positively. The severity of morphologic damage was the best predictor of the number of psychiatric symptoms. Socioeconomic background and social environment had little effect on psychiatric status. The most seriously dysmorphic children had lasting retardation which did not respond to rehabilitative measures, suggesting severe prenatal brain damage. Decreased impairment in the older age groups indicated some capacity for developmental improvement. In a pilot program in Saskatchewan, early intervention was successful in reducing the severity of intellectual deficits in 30 children whose mothers drank heavily during pregnancy (Nanson et al, 1981). The program was primarily home based but was supplemented with visits to a central clinic. Therapists concentrated on teaching parents techniques to stimulate the children at home.

Learning and behavioral disorders were observed in two boys who had been exposed to large amounts of alcohol in utero (Shaywitz et al, 1981). Both had midfacial anomalies, but, atypically, had large heads and neither prenatal nor postnatal growth failure. Their cognitive/linguistic/pragmatic abilities were the most impaired. Scores were within the borderline retarded range on verbal tests of intelligence but were average or above on nonverbal tests. Early developmental delay in language acquisition and use, as well as hypervigilance, distractibility, and anxiety were evident. Participation in special education programs with individualized instruction, consistent routines, limited visual and auditory distractions, speech therapy, and parent training proved beneficial. Followup evaluations confirmed steady gains in all aspects of development (Shaywitz et al, 1982). Since these two boys did not meet diagnostic criteria for FAS, alcohol's role in their developmental delays has been questioned (Miller, 1982; Valente, 1982; Farber, 1982). However, the authors defended their conclusions on the basis of specific language and cognitive dysfunction. While case reports leave many questions unanswered, they can stimulate further investigation of the specificity of linguistic, cognitive, and behavioral disorders.

Sleep

The organization of sleep in neonates exposed to high BACs during fetal life has been investigated by several methods. Sleep states on the third day of life were observed for a 24-hour period by means of a continuous nonintrusive bassinet sleep monitor, and for one interfeed interval by standard sleep polygraphy (Sander et al, 1977). Measures of the infants' sleep states obtained from the bassinet sleep monitor had a high correlation with standard polygraphic determination of REM and non-REM states. Fourteen infants whose mothers drank heavily throughout pregnancy were more restless, with more frequent major body movements and more quiet sleep periods interrupted by awake states than nine babies whose mothers were moderate or rare drinkers, and eight infants whose mothers reduced alcohol consumption before the third trimester (Rosett et al, 1979). Differences were dose related: the greater the alcohol consumption in the third trimester had been, the less time the infant slept. Followup studies should differentiate acute physiologic CNS changes due to intoxication and withdrawal from chronic alterations in brain function. However, even transient disturbances during the neonatal period could indirectly alter later behavior by having a detrimental effect on the quality of mother–infant interaction. A baby with an erratic sleep schedule is demanding for the best mother to care for. When the mother is drinking heavily and has a limited tolerance for frustration, it seriously hampers the development of satisfying attachments between mother and child.

Disturbances in reaching and maintaining quiet sleep were observed in two-hour sleep polygraphy studies of 34 infants born to alcoholic mothers (Havlicek and Childiaeva, 1982). Dose-dependent increases in EEG hypersynchrony were detected during active REM sleep with values exceeding those of healthy infants by more than 200%. Differences persisted for six weeks. The babies also showed more restlessness, limb jerks, and general body movements. Their birthweights were significantly lower than controls. Offspring of women who had been drinking at least 2 oz AA on some occasions and who reported that they stopped drinking during pregnancy demonstrated less EEG hypersynchrony than infants whose mothers had continued to drink. Further analysis revealed that maternal smoking had no effect on infant EEG (Chernick et al, 1983). The effects of lower doses of alcohol on infant sleep were investigated by naturalistic observations of 124 one-day-old infants (Landesman-Dwyer et al, 1978). No differences in REM sleep were found in the children of moderate drinkers, although there was decreased body activity and more time with eyes open.

Evoked potentials

Hrbek et al (1982) found that evoked responses in 25 neonates with alcohol abusing mothers (MAA) differed from those of 37 SGA infants and 25 controls. The brain's responses to auditory, visual, and somatosensory stimuli can be investigated by the electroencephalographic recording of evoked potentials. This provides an index of maturation and function of subcortical structures in the early period of life, when few or no neurological symptoms are present. Abnormal response patterns to visual stimuli were observed in 25% of the MAA neonates, 2.7% of the SGA babies, and none of the controls. Similarly, distinct somatosensory abnormalities were elicited in 56% of the MAA infants, 37% of the SGA group, and 4% of the controls. Followup evaluations demonstrated prolonged brainstem transmission time for auditory evoked responses in three MAA infants at ages ranging from 7 to 30 months.

Changes in brainstem auditory evoked potentials in rat pups prenatally exposed to alcohol are consistent with the findings on infants
(Church and Holloway, 1980). Prolonged auditory transmission
time was observed in alcohol-exposed pups examined periodically
from 2 to 10 weeks of age. Differences diminished but did not disappear with age. Although there was catch-up growth, hearing loss
persisted. The authors suggest that this may reflect deficient myelination or impaired synaptic function.

Fetal breathing

Alcohol has been associated with decreased fetal breathing. Following oral administration of 1 oz of vodka to the mothers, Fox et al
(1978) observed periods of apnea of 50 minutes or more in each of
seven exposed fetuses. Lewis and Boylan (1979) administered a similar dose and observed a reduction in fetal breathing movements
from 46% to 14% of the test period. The clinical implications of these
findings are unclear since fetal oxygen is supplied via the placenta
and is not dependent on in utero breathing activity (see Chapter 3).
However, alcohol's interference with breathing movements in utero
may be a sensitive indicator of depression of CNS regulatory
mechanisms. Alcohol may impair the ability of lung and respiratory
muscles to function postpartum through changes in surfactant, a
surface-active agent in fetal lungs which prevents collapse of alveoli
after birth. Sokol et al (1983) observed abnormal surfactant in neonates of heavy drinkers. Collapse of alveoli after birth can cause
anoxia which is associated with cerebral palsy and mental retardation (Stechler and Halton, 1982).

Mukherjee and Hodgen (1982) observed a spasm of the uterine
artery in monkeys following intravenous injection of very large volumes of alcohol within 1–2 minutes. Fifteen minutes after infusion
of a dose equivalent to 3 g/kg of maternal weight, BACs reached
250 mg percent. The spasm coincided with peak BACs, with recovery noticed at 30 minutes. The authors suggested that this "striking
interruption of feto-placental circulation may explain one of the
mechanisms of mental retardation" associated with FAS. However,
the dose of alcohol that was used was excessively high and the conditions under which it was administered do not approximate human
consumption (Joffe, 1983). The human equivalent would be to

inject the alcohol contained in 36 drinks of 80 proof whiskey into the femoral vein of a 60 kg woman in her 32nd week of pregnancy (Kimball, 1983). The acute effect on the uterine artery probably resulted from local irritation caused by the bolus of alcohol. Altura et al (1983) observed concentration-dependent contractions when ethanol was added to isolated human umbilical arteries and veins. No effects were seen in arteries below the threshold concentration of 52 mg percent or in veins below 86 mg percent. Considerable degrees of contraction occurred with BACs of 220–310 mg percent. Contractions peaked within 4–10 minutes and continued until alcohol was removed. Findings from these studies suggest that chronic intoxication throughout gestation produces umbilical-placental constriction with concomitant fetal damage.

CNS abnormalities

NEUROPATHOLOGY

Neuropathological observations of four human brains exposed in utero to high concentrations of alcohol revealed gross structural abnormalities (Clarren et al, 1978). Three subjects died neonatally; one was a stillborn fetus. The diagnosis of FAS was confirmed in two of them. The most frequent findings were leptomeningeal neuroglial heterotopia, sheets of aberrant neural and glial tissue covering part of the brain surface. In two cases, hydrocephalus was observed. The similarity of these abnormalities suggested that the CNS had been vulnerable during early stages of organogenesis. However a broader period of CNS vulnerability to the teratogenic effects of alcohol was suggested by autopsies of three other children and three fetuses (Peiffer et al, 1979). All had been exposed to high concentrations of alcohol in utero. The three postnatal cases were severely dysmorphic and met the criteria for diagnosing FAS. A spectrum of brain malformations were observed: heterotopias, hydrocephalus internus, agenesis of corpus collosum, microdisplasia, and hydranencephaly. In mice, dogs, and miniature swine, gross neuroanatomical defects including hydrocephaly, exencephaly, microcephaly, and absent corpus collosum have been described following exposure in utero to high blood alcohol concentrations (Kronick, 1976; Chernoff, 1977; Randall and Taylor, 1979; Dexter et al, 1980; Ellis and Pick, 1980; Bannigan and Burke, 1982).

FACE–BRAIN DYSMORPHOLOGY

Facial development begins during the early weeks of gestation, in close approximation to brain development. Exposure to a high dose of alcohol at a critical stage of embryogenesis (around the 50th day of human gestation) may disrupt organization of the face and CNS. Small brain size is associated with early closure of growth areas, shortening of the anterior base of the skull, and reduced forward growth of the face. Cephalometric radiographs revealed significant differences in skull and face measurements between 12 FAS cases and controls (Frias et al, 1982). Abnormalities included shortening of the anterior cranial base, retrusion of the maxilla, and shortened posterior height. Contrary to clinical impressions, maxillary and mandibular lengths were normal.

When evaluating facial dysmorphology, the skill of the examiner is particularly critical. Among children whose facial characteristics are most severely affected, identification is relatively easy. Among mildly affected children, many features approach the normal range of variability, are less specific, and more difficult to diagnose as FAS. The neonate face served as a clear marker only in the Seattle study, where pairs of infants were compared. In the other studies, when a whole range of infants were viewed on a particular day, the examining pediatricians had difficulty identifying neonates who exhibited FAS features. Differentiation may require special training in dysmorphology. The diagnostic value of these signs is diminished if they cannot easily be identified by practicing pediatricians.

Patient age may also be a factor in the identification of dysmorphology. At Boston City Hospital facial features were identified more easily among older children than among neonates. Others have reported that with further growth, particularly when children enter adolescence, the facial signs may again become ambiguous, except in the most severely affected patients (Lemoine et al, 1968; Seidenberg and Majewski, 1978).

Facial anomalies were observed in a group of newborn rhesus monkeys exposed to alcohol in one of three regimens starting on gestational day 21 (Altshuler et al, in press). Doses ranging from 2.5–5.0 g/kg per day were administered either continuously or episodically. The neonates had flat faces and low-set ears. Cranial length, cranial height, and length of the cranial base were diminished. The angles of the mandibular, maxillary, and chin were larger. Facial dysmorphology was seen in association with low birth weight and other morphologic and behavioral abnormalities. At 12 months, the morphologic differences disappeared but the intellectual and behavioral deficits persisted (Altshuler, personal communication).

Neurologic, developmental, and facial abnormalities were observed in pigtailed macaque monkeys exposed to alcohol in utero (Clarren and Bowden, 1982). Alcohol treatment was equivalent to binges of 6 and 10 standard drinks. Effects were found to be dose-dependent. In the offspring of one monkey fed 4.1 g/kg once a week from 40 days after conception to term, the brain was 30% smaller than normal and grossly dysplastic. Cortical organization was abnormal in the frontal, parietal, and occipital lobes. At 6 months, the monkey had a short and retrusive maxilla, wide nose, flat philtrum, and small posteriorly rotated ears. Audiovisual response and activity were retarded and motor development was delayed. There was neither growth retardation nor malformations of other organs. One animal exposed to 2.5 g/kg weekly was less severely affected. The brain showed small leptomeningeal neuroglial heterotopias and neuronal fallout with gliosis in the superficial cortical layers in the frontal lobes. The lateral geniculate was small and dysplastic. There was no facial dysmorphology. Neonatal assessments at 10 days were normal, as was motor development. The offspring of a second monkey fed 2.5 g/kg weekly was normal and displayed no developmental abnormalities.

Sulik and Johnston (1982) have experimentally produced facial malformations similar to those observed in FAS. C57 mice embryos treated with ethanol on gestational day 9 showed marked deficiency in the size of the neural plate, particularly in the forebrain, with concomitant facial dysmorphology. Mouse fetuses exposed to two large doses of alcohol on gestational day 7 demonstrated retarded brain growth and abnormal facial features within 48 hours (Sulik and Johnston, 1983). Peak blood alcohol levels of 195 mg percent followed the first injection and 218 mg percent the second. The dysmorphogenesis was similar to that observed clinically. Effects varied when exposure times differed by only 4 hours (Sulik et al, 1981). When treatment was initiated at 6 days 20 hours, the highest number of gross craniofacial malformations and fewest resorptions occurred. Treatment at 7 days 0 hours yielded fewer abnormalities but the highest number of FAS-like cranio-facial features. The group treated at 7 days 4 hours demonstrated the lowest number of abnormalities but the highest resorption incidence. In a similar study, brain abnormalities followed exposure on days 7 and 8 (Webster et al, 1980). Exposure on days 9 through 11 caused limb abnormalities but no change in brain growth or structure, suggesting that the nature of the defect depends on the period of development. Day 7 represents a developmental stage comparable to the third gestational week in humans. Abnormalities were produced when alcohol levels of at least 400 mg percent were achieved. The lower blood alcohol figures reported by Sulik et al were derived from breath alcohol levels.

BRAIN STRUCTURE AND SIZE

Microcephaly, head circumference below the third percentile, is one of the diagnostic signs of FAS. Since head size expands to accommodate the brain, microcephaly reflects a small brain and is commonly associated with mental retardation. Brain growth has been retarded in fetal and neonatal experimental animals in association with doses of alcohol in the range of 35% of calories supplied as ethanol (Volk, 1977; Hofteig and Druse, 1978; Jacobson et al, 1978). This represents a dose level in rats of 6–7 g/kg per day of ethanol. A human who consumes 35% of calories as ethanol is a chronic alcoholic. No observable growth or behavioral effects have resulted from doses in the range of 1–2 g/kg per day (Abel, 1980a; Sonderegger et al, 1982; Randall, 1982). Initial studies of the effects of alcohol on brain growth, structure, and neurochemistry were conducted with large doses to investigate any potential effects. Later studies have analyzed the effects of specific doses and developmental stage of exposure.

The vulnerability of the CNS may be greatest during periods of rapid brain growth. In humans, the developing brain has two growth spurts. The first occurs during the first trimester. The second begins during the third trimester and continues for the first 18 months of life. Rats are born with less mature brains; their second period of rapid brain growth occurs postnatally. When ethanol was administered to newborn rat pups via intragastric cannulae in doses sufficient to maintain inebriation, total brain weight was reduced by 20% even though total body weight did not differ from the control group (Diaz and Samson, 1980). Blood ethanol concentrations within a narrow range were required to produce microcephaly (Samson and Grant, 1983). Doses below 5 g/kg per day did not reduce brain size. Doses between 6 and 6.5 g/kg per day produced microcephaly while doses over 7 g/kg per day caused death.

In addition to the effects of alcohol on the size of the whole brain, changes have been found in specific regions. Since the cerebellum develops later than the cerebral cortex, it is particularly vulnerable during late gestational stages. Cerebellar development and production of Purkinje cells was inhibited in rat pups following postnatal exposure to high peak alcohol levels (Bauer-Moffett and Altman, 1975, 1977; Anderson and Sides, 1978). Comparison of susceptibility during fetal, neonatal, and adult life demonstrated that the Purkinje cells were most sensitive in the neonatal period (Phillips and Cragg, 1982). Cerebellar weights were reduced by 12% in 21 day old rats exposed to alcohol throughout gestation and until day 21 postpartum (Borges and Lewis, 1982). Alcohol levels reached 135 mg/dl in maternal blood and 44 mg/dl in neonatal blood. Body weights and whole brain weights did not differ from controls. A subsequent study demonstrated that alcohol at this level reduced the granule cell population of the internal granular layer but did not affect Purkinje cells (Borges and Lewis, 1983).

Kornguth et al (1979) observed s   cerebellar and cerebral weights in ethanol-exposed rat pup brains examined at 11 or 14 days postnatal. Although body weights were also lower, brain tissue appeared to be selectively disadvantaged. Abnormal cerebellar development was characterized by a reduction in cerebellar mass, an increase in the external granule cell layer, and reduced enzymatic activity. There was also a reduction in the level of serum thyroxine in alcohol-exposed pups. Other drugs such as methadone, as well as prenatal stress and malnutrition, may also cause delayed cerebellar maturation by reducing serum thyroxine at critical periods.

In utero exposure to ethanol results in multiple abnormalities at the cellular level in the fetal brain. Brain growth may reflect an increase in cell number (hyperplasia) or in cell size (hypertrophy). This can be differentiated by measuring DNA, RNA, lipids, and proteins. Since the DNA content of each cell is a constant, and protein, lipid, and RNA content increase with cell size, the ratios of these other components to DNA can be used as a measure of cell size.

A decrease in the number of total brain cells as well as cell size was deduced from the ratio of protein to DNA in alcohol-exposed sheep fetuses delivered 10 days before term (Potter et al, 1980). A reduction in brain weight was accompanied by a significant reduction of both brain DNA and protein. Dams had been fed 10% ethanol solution in quantities sufficient to produce intoxication and addiction throughout gestation. In addition to the adverse effects on the brain, there were reductions in size and weight of the fetal body as a whole and of the visceral organs. A reduction in the number of fetal brain cells has also occurred in rats exposed to high concentrations of ethanol (Woodson and Ritchey, 1979). Acute alcohol exposure on gestational days 14–16 resulted in significant (6%) reduction in net DNA in rat brains (Henderson et al, 1979). Exposure on days 11–13 had no effect on net brain DNA although there were reductions in other organs. Chronic ethanol exposure caused a decrease in net DNA only in kidneys.

Neuroanatomic study of the hippocampus demonstrates that alcohol in utero can disturb microscopic brain structure in the absence of gross malformations. When maternal rats were fed liquid diets containing 35% ethanol-derived calories, their pups had abnormally distributed mossy fibers in temporal regions of the hippocampus (West et al, 1981). These fibers represent the major output from granule cells. Histologic study of hippocampal pyramidal cells revealed a marked reduction in the extent of basilar dendrites (Davies and Smith, 1981). Ethanol had been administered as 25% of daily calories to maternal mice during late pregnancy and the first postpartum week.

Restitution

The observed alterations in neonatal brain size and structure may not be permanent (Volk et al, 1981). Offspring of rats, fed 37% of daily calories as alcohol, were killed at ages ranging from 3 to 21 days postpartum. Morphologic analysis of the cerebellar Purkinje cells revealed significantly smaller nuclei on day 7. At days 12 and 17 there were no differences, suggesting that alcohol caused a developmental delay with a potential for recovery when alcohol was no longer present. Delays in cortical development were also observed among offspring of rats fed a modified Freund diet with 30% of calories derived from ethanol (Jacobson et al, 1978). At 14 days postnatal, complete cortical lamination was apparent in controls but not in the alcohol-exposed pups. At 23 days, however, complete cortical lamination was observed in the alcohol-exposed pups.

In mice, cell necrosis affecting the neuroepithelium both in the closed caudal portion of the neural tube and the unclosed cranial neural tube was observed six hours after ethanol exposure (Bannigan and Burke, 1982). At 24 hours post exposure, the neuroepithelium showed signs of repair. At 50 hours, the neuroepithelium was completely clear of debris resulting from cell necrosis, although some embryos had open neural tube defects and some had been resorbed. Many fetuses survived to day 19 with no apparent gross defects, demonstrating varied capacity to repair.

Acetaldehyde's teratogenic effects on the developing CNS may also be reversible. Neural tube defects and retarded growth were observed on gestational day 10 in rat embryos exposed in vivo to acetaldehyde on days 6, 7, 8, or 9 (O'Shea and Kaufman, 1981). The neuroepithelium was atypical in appearance with irregular cell surface and spiny intercellular processes. The location of the defect along the neuraxis was related to the developmental stage at time of exposure. Following injection on day 7, hindbrain (70%), midbrain (20%), and neural tube (10%) defects were seen on day 10. The incidence of neural tube defects observed on day 12 was considerably lower (2%) with no increase in the incidence of resorption. The lowered incidence of neural tube defects led the authors to suggest that compensation or reversibility occurs.

Neurochemistry

A complete understanding of the effects of alcohol on the fetal and adult CNS requires investigating the neurochemical mechanisms that pass signals between neurons by releasing neurotransmitters at specific synapses. Alterations in the release and re-uptake of neurotransmitters, as well as changes in the synaptic membrane receptor sites have been demonstrated. Some neurochemical changes may persist and alter functions throughout life.

The most investigated neurotransmitters are the catecholamines: norepinephrine, serotonin, and dopamine. After experimental exposure to alcohol, catecholamine levels have been reported to be both elevated (Rawat, 1977) and decreased (Lau et al, 1976; Detering et al, 1980a). The inconsistencies may have resulted from various methodological differences, including dose, time, and route of alcohol administration, nutrition, animal age at time of testing, and the study of brain areas or whole brain. Chemical analysis of discrete brain regions has revealed changes which were not found in studies of the whole brain. Neurochemistry is a young and rapidly developing field, and carefully designed studies promise a better understanding of the effects of alcohol on the CNS and behavior.

Rat pups continuously exposed to ethanol as 30–40% of total caloric intake demonstrated deficiencies in adrenal catecholamines and adrenal-beta-hydroxylase activity (Lau et al, 1976). Both parameters returned to normal when alcohol was withdrawn, suggesting reversible retardation in the maturation of adrenal catecholamine stores.

The activity levels of brain enzymes involved in synthesizing catecholamine neurotransmitters were altered in three-week-old pups exposed to ethanol prenatally and postnatally (Detering et al, 1979). Maternal rats were fed a regular stock diet, a high-dose liquid diet containing 35% of the calories as ethanol, and a pair-fed diet with maltose-dextrin substituted for the calories supplied by ethanol. Body growth and brain growth were retarded in both groups fed the liquid diet. However, the offspring of high-dose ethanol-fed dams showed greater retardation in all growth and brain-size indices. The enzyme activity of tyrosine hydroxylase was increased by both prenatal and postnatal alcohol exposure; dopamine beta hydroxylase activity increased following prenatal exposure but decreased after postnatal administration. At three weeks of age the norepinephrine (NE) levels in the hypothalamus of rats exposed pre- or postnatally was 30–60% lower than levels in control pups (Detering et al, 1980c). Significantly lower NE levels were found in the hypothalamus of six-month-old rats which had been exposed to ethanol prenatally but were given regular lab chow after weaning (Detering et al, 1980a). The decreased NE levels seem to be due to an increased rate of NE removal and not a decrease in synthesis (Detering et al, 1980b).

Ethanol and malnutrition alter separate components of the catecholamine neurotransmission system. In another study, blood ethanol concentrations were associated with decreases in whole brain levels of norepinephrine, dopamine, and serotonin in newborn rat pups (Shoemaker et al, 1983). Blood ethanol concentrations ranged from 93–274 mg/dl. Dietary composition affected BACs. Deficits were found to be a consequence of ethanol in the diet rather than of undernutrition. Levels of the peptide neurotransmitter, beta endorphin, also showed a striking dose-related increase in the midbrain and hindbrain of newborn pups exposed to alcohol in utero.

Myelination—the development of the lipo-protein sheath surrounding many axons—is necessary for transmission of signals. Alcohol's effects on myelin formation have been investigated in rat pups of ethanol-fed mothers and pair-fed controls. When dams were fed ethanol for one month before conception and during gestation, their offspring demonstrated a premature onset and slowdown of active CNS myelination (Druse and Hofteig, 1977). When ethanol was administered only during gestation, CNS myelination was near normal at birth. However at 53 days of age, the ethanol-exposed pups had an excess of the chemically and morphologically immature heavy coat (Hofteig and Druse, 1978). In addition to changes in myelination, alterations in the content of glycoproteins and gangliosides within the synaptic plasma membranes of rat pup brains have been reported following chronic exposure throughout pregnancy (Druse et al, 1981). Brief exposure during the third trimester had no effect.

In humans, preputial tissue, readily available from circumcision of neonates, permits nerve fibers to be examined. Altered myelination of peripheral nerves was found in the prepuces of four newborns whose mothers drank at least 45 drinks a month with five or more on some occasions (Amankwah et al, 1982). Pathologic findings included unmyelinated nerve fibers with increased vesicular and tubular elements of agranular endoplasmic reticulum.

Neuroendocrine function

The interrelationships between the hypothalamus, the pituitary, the other endocrine glands and target organs have suggested a single neuroendocrine system with multiple axes. Taylor et al (1981, 1983) studied pituitary-adrenal response to stress in rats exposed to ethanol from day 8 to parturition. Maternal ethanol intake averaged 12 g/kg per day with BACs of 63.7 mg/dl at 09.00 hours and 128.2 mg/dl at 20.00 hours. At birth the fetal alcohol exposed pups tended to weigh less than pair-fed controls, although the differences were not significant. The plasma and brain corticosterone levels of pups killed on the first day of life were significantly higher than those in the pair-fed controls. Adults which had been exposed to alcohol in utero showed significantly higher corticosterone levels when subjected to stress by four different methods: intraperitoneal injection of alcohol; cardiac puncture; exposure to cold (4°C) for 60 minutes; and 30 minutes of intermittent noise and cage shaking. Other measures of adult pituitary-adrenal activity in the rat were not affected by exposure to alcohol in utero.

Nelson et al (1983) also observed alterations in reaction to stress. Fetal alcohol exposed adult rats did not differ from controls in their voluntary consumption of 7% alcohol and water when they were housed under standard laboratory conditions. They did not differ during a week of chronic stress induced by administering shocks to their feet. For 2 weeks after the chronic stress, however, fetal alcohol exposed animals consumed significantly more alcohol and water than controls. McGivern et al (1984) found no differences in preference for ethanol between fetal alcohol exposed rats and pair-fed controls. Met- and Leu-enkephalin levels were significantly elevated in the globus pallidus of the adult fetal alcohol exposed animals whereas pituitary levels were unaffected. Differences in endogenous opioid levels may be related to differences in response to stress.

Augmented stress-induced corticosterone responses result from a persistent alteration in the central neural mechanisms that regulate hypothalamic-pituitary-adrenal function. The lack of appropriate neuroendocrine response inhibition is analogous to the behavioral defects observed by Riley et al (1979a,b). They may be linked to the effects on brain catecholamines, particularly the norepinephrine levels resported by Detering and the neuroanatomic changes in the hippocampus observed by West.

In many higher vertebrates, sexual differentiation of reproductive and behavior patterns is affected by the induction of permanent and essentially irreversible sex differences in CNS function in response to gonadal hormones secreted early in development (MacLusky and Naftolin, 1981). Kakihana et al (1980) studied the brains of 1–2 day old male rats whose mothers had received 35% of their total calories as ethanol. Compared with the offspring of rats pair-fed isocaloric sucrose, dihydrotestosterone levels were lower in the brains of the male pups and corticosterone concentrations were higher in the brains of both sexes. There was also a tendency towards reduced testicular weight and increased adrenal weight among ethanol-exposed neonatal male rats. Rats' preference for a saccharine flavored liquid diet is sexually dimorphic and highly sensitive to alterations of androgens (but not estrogen levels) during the perinatal period. McGivern (personal communication) found that prenatal consumption of liquid diets containing 36% of the total calories as ethanol can abolish the sexual differences in this normally dimorphic behavior.

The effects of differences in prenatal endocrine stimulation on human development and sexual behavior are less clear (Ehrhardt and Meyer-Bahlburg, 1979). Retarded sexual maturation has been suggested by the late opening of the vagina in mice and rats following in utero exposure to large doses of alcohol (Boggan et al, 1979; Tittmar, 1977). Case reports of genitourinary malformations in FAS children may reflect androgen deficiency in utero. Delayed menarche has been reported in adolescent daughters of alcoholic mothers who drank heavily during pregnancy (Shurygin, 1974; Robe et al, 1979). Since sexual behavior and dimorphism can be specified and investigated in animal offspring with greater precision than in humans, it represents an important area for future study.

Behavior: experimental models

The specificity of behavioral effects of in utero alcohol exposure is obscured in humans by the multiple determinants of development, including the continued interaction between the child, the parents, and the environment. The most consistent clinical observations of alcohol-exposed children are hyperactivity, impulsivity, distractibility, and attentional deficits. Experiments with rats have demonstrated behavioral sequelae of alcohol exposure in utero analogous to those observed clinically. Greater arousal was observed among alcohol-exposed pups in tests of activity including wheel running and Y-maze behavior (Martin et al, 1978; Osborne et al, 1980). Heightened exploratory behaviors (nose poking and head dipping) occurred in a dose-dependent manner (Riley et al, 1979c). In open field activity, no differences were found at doses of 1–2 g/kg body weight (Abel and York, 1979; Sonderegger et al, 1982) but at higher doses (6 g/kg/day) differences were observed (Abel, 1979a). Prenatally exposed pups were more active than pair-fed controls early in life but the differences disappeared with maturation (Shaywitz et al, 1976; Bond and DiGiusto, 1977). Diminished response inhibition was found in alcohol-exposed rats in tests of spontaneous alternation, reversal learning, and passive avoidance extinction (Riley et al, 1979a,b). Further testing of impaired response inhibition differentially reinforced low rates of responding in such a way that the animals had to learn to inhibit responding for a 10 second period. Alcohol-related differences in learning to withhold response were more apparent at maturity (70 days) than during earlier testing (Driscoll et al, 1980).

Critical reviews of the experimental literature concur that although various methodologies affect the results of specific studies, overall trends have emerged (Bond, 1981; Abel, 1982b; Randall, 1982; Riley, 1982). Prenatal ethanol in sufficient doses causes delays in maturation of behavioral, motor, and cognitive capacities. There are no observable effects with low doses (1–2 g/kg per day). The magnitude of the effect increases with dose (Abel, 1980a, 1982a; Randall, 1982). Activity levels and learning ability are altered. These are age related and frequently disappear over time. Bond (1981) identified a consistent pattern of activity in 12 experimental studies. Rats exposed in utero to alcohol doses greater than 6–7 g/kg per day exhibited increased activity prior to age 70 days in comparison with control offspring. A review of ten studies of learning ability revealed dose-related differences in performance that were dependent on activity level. Performance was enhanced in tasks that required increased activity and impaired in tasks requiring low levels of activity. In the latter, performance improved when activity lessened with maturity. When tasks did not depend on activity, learning deficits persisted. Riley (1982) has also observed that age-related improvements in learning tasks reflect changes in activity level and response inhibition rather than changes in cognitive deficits.

Summary

Consumption of large amounts of alcohol can affect several systems in the developing brain and alter structure, neurochemistry, and function. Intelligence, activity, and sleep regulation are adversely affected by in utero exposure to high doses of alcohol. The nature and extent of the abnormalities are related to blood alcohol levels and the gestational stage of exposure. No clinically significant behaviors have been reported to be affected by consumption levels in the range of 1 oz AA per day.

Severe facial dysmorphology and retardation probably reflect markedly abnormal brain anatomy. In both clinical and experimental programs, restitution and reversibility have been observed. The behavioral consequences of anatomical alterations are the least responsive to remedial programs; however, behavioral aberrations that reflect developmental delays lessen with maturation and seem to benefit from remedial programs.

Seven

Methodologic Issues

During the last ten years knowledge about the adverse effects of ethanol on the fetus has expanded rapidly, and research has been conducted by scientists in many disciplines. Results of well over a thousand clinical, epidemiological, and experimental studies have been reported, often with contradictory findings and conclusions. Methodologic differences in study design have resulted in inconsistencies. Research on alcohol's effects is subject to ethical and pragmatic constraints inherent in working with human subjects. In addition, many inconsistencies have been ignored, and data has been selectively cited and interpreted (Abel, 1982b). As a result, the danger of small amounts of alcohol has been exaggerated. There is confusion among health care providers about what is appropriate advice to give to pregnant women. While it is tempting to wait until definitive answers are available, clinical situations demand decisions, and these decisions must be based on current knowledge (Rosett and Weiner, 1980). In this chapter we discuss methodologic issues in fetal alcohol research and their relevance to clinical decisions.

Defining risk levels of maternal drinking

The foremost clinical dilemma is to precisely determine dangerous levels of alcohol consumption. Prospective and retrospective studies have attempted to investigate dose levels associated with adverse effects. However, there is no consensus on a precise dose-response relationship. Methods for obtaining and interpreting data on maternal drinking patterns vary from study to study. All have relied on self-reports, but different methods have been used to obtain them. Definitions of "a drink" and of drinking patterns have not been standardized. Associations found in one study between a level of drinking and outcome may be denied by another simply because levels have been defined and labelled differently.

ASSESSING DRINKING PATTERNS

The use of self-reports introduces a degree of uncertainty into research on dose-response. Self-reported histories of alcohol consumption are rarely accurate. Differences between actual and reported behavior can be caused by memory problems, social pressure for acceptable responses, misreporting, and guilt about illness (Sudman and Bradburn, 1974). The accuracy of self-reports can be further affected by methodologic variables, including timing, setting, and question format. In relational research, the validity of individual responses is critical. In analyzing outcome, errors of over or underreporting do not average out, but become additive.

The timing of the interview is one of the most critical methodologic issues in obtaining valid personal drinking histories. Reports of recent drinking are more reliable than reports of earlier drinking, which may in fact reflect recent patterns (Fitzgerald and Mulford, 1978). As time passes, approximate measures of consumption are more reliable than precise accounts (Little et al, 1977). Responses to questions about alcohol consumption obtained during pregnancy differ from retrospective reports. During pregnancy, concern for the health of the baby helps motivate the woman to respond honestly. Once the baby is born, fear of censure for past drinking behavior may influence her to deny alcohol use, especially if abnormalities have been observed in the neonate.

The impact of timing may be inferred from our study at Boston City Hospital. When 327 women were interviewed both prenatally and postpartum, heavy drinking during pregnancy was reported three times more often in the prenatal interview (Hingson et al, 1982). The Boston experience should be considered when analyzing data obtained retrospectively, and the tendency to underreport should be acknowledged. In Loma Linda, alcohol use during pregnancy was described postpartum by all study participants (Kuzma and Kissinger, 1981). The number (1.5%) who reported drinking 2 or more drinks per day during pregnancy was relatively low compared with surveys of drinking patterns among pregnant women. The authors appropriately discuss the women's drinking patterns according to their relative ranking within the distribution of alcohol intake for the entire study population. Adverse fetal outcomes were associated with the 3% who drank most frequently, but no attempt was made to define the amount of alcohol consumed (Kuzma and Sokol, 1982).

Biases of setting and timing may have influenced reports of drinking in Kline et al's (1980) study of spontaneous abortions. Frequent alcohol consumption was reported more often by 616 women who suffered abortions than by age-matched controls. When consumption of at least 1 oz AA was reported, the risk of abortion increased in direct relation to the frequency of consumption. The accuracy of the self-reports was questioned in an editorial published in Lancet concurrently with the paper (Alcohol and Spontaneous Abortion, 1980). Women who had suffered an abortion were interviewed on the hospital ward, whereas the controls were seen in the prenatal clinic. The experience of miscarriage and the subsequent hospitalization may have heightened the women's awareness of their health habits and increased their reports of alcohol consumption. In addition, questions about drinking pertained to a longer time period for the controls than for the cases, since interviews were conducted later in pregnancy. Their responses could have been biased by impaired recall, or could have reflected recent alcohol consumption, which has been shown to be less frequent during pregnancy (Stein and Kline, 1983).

Retrospective reports of alcohol consumed during a pregnancy years earlier are particularly vulnerable to bias. Recovering alcoholics who celebrate the anniversary of their abstinence in Alcoholics Anonymous meetings are accurate about the date of their last drink, but may be less certain of the exact quantities they consumed while they were drinking heavily. Most women are no more likely to be able to precisely recall their consumption after a month has elapsed than they would be able to remember exactly what they ate. Only exceptional occasions are recalled. These biases may affect data demonstrating relationships between birthweights and drinking patterns of alcoholics, abstinent alcoholics, and controls which was gathered an average of 7½ years after delivery (Little and Streissguth, 1978).

The format of the questions may also influence responses. Underestimates tend to occur when women are asked about alcohol use in vague or general terms. In a national study of American drinking practices, Cahalan et al (1969) found that separate questions about each beverage elicited more accurate information than global questions about drinking. In addition, questions about average alcohol consumption do not provide information about occasions when large amounts are consumed. The study by Harlap and Shiono (1980) focused on the relationship between birth control and reproductive outcome. Women were asked about their "average" daily consumption of "alcoholic beverages" rather than specifically about the frequency, quantity, and variability in their use of beer, wine, and liquor. A dose-response relationship was observed between average alcohol consumed and spontaneous abortions: the relative risk was 1 : 98 for women whose average was 1–2 drinks a day and 3 : 53 for women who averaged more than three drinks a day. The authors qualified their findings, stating, "Our data do not enable us . . . to assess whether there was any significant degree of underreporting." Sokol (1980) observed that associations occurred only among the heaviest drinking 2.9% of the population. Extrapolating from other studies of alcohol use among pregnant women, he suggested that the low levels of alcohol consumption claimed by these women do indeed represent underreporting.

Biases may result from individual variations in defining a drink. At Boston City Hospital, discussions about the amount of alcohol consumed in a drink revealed that heavy drinkers frequently understated quantities. Some reported an 8 oz tumbler full of liquor as one drink. Studies that have assumed that all reported servings were of equal size (Hingson et al, 1982; Kuzma and Kissinger, 1981; Harlap and Shiono, 1980) may have underestimated consumption levels of the heaviest drinkers.

Assessment of alcohol use may improve with repeated inquiry. Single interviews identify current practices but miss changes in drinking patterns commonly observed among pregnant women. Some women always discuss alcohol use in the past tense. For them, the full pattern only emerges with repeated interviews. However, multiple inquiries may produce discrepant responses resulting from changes in reporting style rather than in actual drinking habits. At Boston City Hospital, behavioral change was validated by the differences in growth patterns between children of women who did and did not report reduction of heavy drinking (Rosett et al, 1983b).

In future studies, efforts should be made to incorporate biochemical techniques to validate drinking histories. Polich (1982) used a breatholizer test and compared actual BACs with reports of recent consumption among alcoholics. Self-reported consumption was underreported at a rate of 25%. The highest rate of underreporting (42%) occurred among individuals who said they had two or fewer drinks on drinking days. Among those who said they consumed 2–8 drinks per day, 30% underreported. Less than 10% of individuals who said that they averaged over 8 drinks a day were underreporting. Self reports of abstention were quite valid.

Established objective measures of alcohol in the blood, breath, urine, or saliva detect only recent drinking. A new sweat-patch test can differentiate those who drink no alcohol from those who consume an average of 1.5 oz AA daily, either continuously or episodically (Phillips and McAloon, 1980). It can be used to assess alcohol consumption over a week's time in cooperative subjects; however, further clinical testing is necessary to assure its reliability and validity. Another objective, integrated time-dose measurement of alcohol consumption may eventually be achieved with a recently identified and apparently specific glycosylated hemoglobin component of erythrocite lysates (Hoberman, 1979; Hoberman and Chiodo, 1982). Barrison et al (1982) measured levels of gamma-glutamyl transpeptidase which rise in response to alcohol. The test was of little value in detecting alcohol abuse among pregnant women because of the physiologic changes that occur regularly during pregnancy. In the absence of biochemical markers, self-reports can be compared with collateral reports obtained from significant others. When drinking is hidden, however, it may also be concealed from family members and friends.

The problems inherent in using self-reports to assess maternal drinking patterns are an obstacle to associating fetal outcome with precise doses of alcohol. It is likely that actual intake is higher than that reported. However, the limits on precision do not preclude associating adverse fetal outcomes with the heaviest drinking women in each population. The rank ordering of drinkers has been shown to be valid (Fitzgerald and Mulford, 1978). Similarly, in test-retests of drinking habits of pregnant women, 71% remained in the same quantity-frequency-variability group although only 24% reported the same AA scores (Little et al, 1977). Overreporting of alcohol use by pregnant women is extremely rare. Heavy drinkers can be differentiated from all others on the basis of reports of high frequency and quantity of alcohol use. At Boston City Hospital, the heavy drinkers reported a mean daily AA score 15 times higher than the moderate (Weiner et al, 1983). High AA scores were also reported by the heavy drinkers in Cleveland (Sokol et al, 1980) and Loma Linda (Kuzma and Kissinger, 1981). In the population as a whole, it has been estimated that 10% of the population consumes 50% of the alcohol (Wuthrich and Hausherr, 1977).

DEFINING DRINKING PATTERNS

In the definition or categorization of drinking patterns, there are three sources of semantic confusion: (1) research groups differ in their use of the same terminology, (2) diverse patterns of quantity, frequency, and variability of drinking are included in one category, and (3) several terms are used by a single research program to define a particular drinking pattern. Differences between definitions of drinking patterns have led to divergent views on the level of drinking associated with adverse effects on the fetus. "Moderate levels" of consumption have been linked to adverse outcomes in studies using classifications we question. Definitions of the heaviest drinking group used by several studies and the percent of women in each population in this group are displayed in Table 7-1. While different terminology is used, each project has differentiated the distinct group of women whose alcohol consumption ranks in the top 2–12% of the study population.

In some studies, women with very different drinking patterns have been grouped together. Little (1977) observed reduced birthweights among children of 20 women who drank more than 1 oz AA per day late in pregnancy. In this study population, she describes four women who would be defined as alcoholics "by any standards." The children of the alcohol-dependent women were not evaluated separately. Kline et al (1980) reported that the "association between spontaneous abortion and drinking during pregnancy,

Table 7-1   Heaviest drinking category as defined in various studies

	SAMPLE SIZE	PERCENT OF WOMEN IN HEAVIEST DRINKING CATEGORY	MINIMUM OZ AA	MEAN OZ AA PER DAY
Boston	1,711	9.4	2.5/occasion	4.6
Cleveland	2,913	11.9	+ MAST[a]	2.0/drinking day
Loma Linda	12,406	1.5	2.0/day	5.9
Paris	9,236	5.5	1.5/day	—
Ottawa	217	3.3	0.85/day	2.5
Seattle	1,529	7.6	1.0/day	—
Northern California	32,019	2.9	0.5/day	—

[a] Michigan Alcoholism Screening Test.

which is evident for drinking as seldom as twice a week . . . becomes stronger with more frequent drinking." If this is so, one would expect that women who drink almost every day would be at higher risk than those who drink two times a week. Unfortunately, these women are grouped together and the outcome for the more frequent drinkers is not differentiated. In both studies, it is impossible to ascertain which problems found within the whole group actually occurred only in the higher drinking subgroup. In a study of mental and motor development at 8 months, decrements were reported among offspring of women who drank more than 1 oz AA per day (Streissguth et al, 1980). Analysis of subgroups demonstrated that decrements only occurred among offspring of the women reporting more than 4 oz AA per day. Similarly, Berkowitz (1981) reported an increased rate of prematurity among women who drank more than 7 drinks a week, but further analysis demonstrated increased incidence only among women consuming at least 14 drinks a week (Berkowitz et al, 1982).

In other analyses, the Seattle research program has used many definitions for drinking groups, scoring responses on alcohol use five ways. Women identified as "heavy" drinkers on one scale were not always considered "heavy" on other scales (Streissguth et al, 1981). Terminology used to describe particular drinking patterns has differed. In the study of mental and motor development at 8 months, women were defined as heavy drinkers if their daily average was more than 1 oz AA (Streissguth et al, 1980). In a four year followup study of a cohort of these infants, women whose daily AA consumption ranged from 1–2.5 oz were defined as moderate social drinkers (Landesman-Dwyer et al, 1981). Women who drank more than 2.5 oz were considered "alcoholic" and removed from the study. Thus women drinking the same amounts were labeled "heavy drinkers" in one study and "moderate social drinkers" in the other.

EXPERIMENTAL MODELS

Dose-response relationships have been tested in animal models in which alcohol consumption and multiple confounding variables can be determined more precisely. However, to extrapolate findings to the clinical situation, the dose tested and the species specificity of outcome factors must be assessed. Differences in alcohol treatment regimens may influence the outcome and subsequent interpretation since nutritional status, blood alcohol levels, and maternal stress are all affected by the route of administration (Abel, 1980b).

When rats are given high doses of alcohol their desire for food decreases. Pair-fed controls help ensure that the observed differences are due to alcohol and not to alcohol-induced undernutrition. Although differences in nutritional intake between experimental and control animals are eliminated by this technique, intestinal malabsorption of nutrients by the experimental group cannot be controlled. Alcohol exposure often causes excessive consumption of water and diarrhea which cause nutritional deficiencies.

Alcohol can be administered experimentally either orally or by injection. Most researchers replace solid chow and water with a vitamin-fortified liquid diet to which specific concentrations of alcohol have been added. Daily caloric and alcohol intake are monitored; control animals are fed equal caloric amounts one day later. Alcohol is sometimes mixed with the drinking water given to experimental animals. However, with this method, high BACs are rarely achieved since few animals drink sufficiently large quantities. Also, precise dose and nutritional intake cannot be controlled.

Intragastric intubation of alcohol is used in species which will not readily ingest alcohol in liquids. Control animals are pair-fed

and intubated with an isocaloric sucrose solution equal in volume
to the administered dose of alcohol. Although it is physiologically
similar to oral ingestion of alcohol, intubation is stressful and high
doses can be fatal.

In small animals such as mice and rats intraperitoneal injections
are used. In monkeys and other large animals, injections are intravenous. Intraperitoneal injection can be stressful to both mother and
fetus. Care must be taken not to puncture the uterus or amniotic
sac. Intravenous injection of concentrated alcohol can cause local
irritation and tissue damage which do not occur with oral ingestion
of even toxic amounts (Wallgren and Barry, 1970). Following injection of high doses, vasoconstriction is apparent in several organ
systems in humans.

No experimental protocol simulates human patterns of consumption and metabolism. Intubation causes high peak levels for brief
periods. Including alcohol in liquid diets causes more gradual fluctuations in BACs with the highest levels occurring during the dark
phase of the dark/light cycle. Alcohol administered by intravenous
injection enters the bloodstream directly. Since it does not pass
through the digestive system, it is not physiologically analogous to
the consumption of beverage alcohol. Also, humans drink in variable
patterns which differ between women and may change from day to
day, unlike the administration of specific doses of alcohol in the
laboratory.

The route of alcohol administration affects the rate of absorption
and resultant peak BACs. Oral doses of 9 g/kg are needed to yield
BACs similar to that achieved by an intraperitoneal dose of 5 g/kg
(Wallgren and Barry, 1970). At lower doses, peak BACs also vary
with route of administration: oral ingestion of 1 g produces a BAC
of 100 mg percent, whereas intraperitoneal injection of 1 g yields a
BAC of 140 mg percent. The composition of the animal's diet can
also affect the BAC (Shoemaker et al, 1983). When rats were fed
diets low in protein, their blood alcohol levels were three times
higher than when fed high protein diets (see Table 7-2).

Alcohol metabolism differs with each species. When extrapolating data from animal to man, it is important to remember that
animals metabolize alcohol at a much faster rate and achieve lower
blood alcohol levels than humans exposed to similar doses. Distribution and equilibration of alcohol following intravenous and
intraperitoneal injections occur in about 30 minutes in mice, less

Table 7-2 Dietary composition and blood ethanol concentration in the rat 4 hours after ingestion

PROTEIN (g/l)	CARBO-HYDRATE (g/l)	ETHANOL (g/l)	BAC (mg/dl)
41.4	24.4	50.0	274.0
90.0	25.3	50.0	92.8

Adapted from Shoemaker et al, 1983.

than an hour in rats, and an hour or more in large animals and man. While rodents metabolize about 300–550 mg/kg/hour, the rate for humans is 100 mg/kg/hour (Wallgren and Barry, 1970).

The BACs used in animal research are often much higher than those found in alcoholics and may even be so high as to be incompatible with life. In man, medullary paralysis may occur at 450 mg/100 ml. Lethal oral doses are 8 g/kg in mice, 9 g/kg in rats, and 5 g/kg for dogs (Wallgren and Barry, 1970). Lethal doses from injection are about half as large.

No unobstrusive methods are available to measure BACs (Abel, 1980b). To obtain accurate levels and determine peak levels and duration of exposure, investigators should test the blood every hour. Since food intake following alcohol ingestion delays absorption and affects the resultant BAC, experimental animals should not be fed following alcohol exposure. Frequent extraction of blood stresses the animal as does permanent insertion of a cannula. Stress itself can affect the offspring's development. Investigators have attempted to avoid stress by testing blood alcohol levels in an independent group of nonpregnant rats. However, pregnancy itself affects blood alcohol levels, reducing the applicability of data from nonpregnant to pregnant animals (Petersen et al, 1977; Abel, 1980b).

Although each experiment produces some information, the animal models also have drawbacks. All information must be considered with recognition of the limitations. When comparing the results of different studies, one must consider whether or not research methodology contributed to inconsistent conclusions. Findings should be evaluated in terms of BACs rather than dose, and the BACs must be assessed to determine whether they are analogous to those in humans.

A consideration of methodologic issues helps define how much alcohol is too much. The relationship between adverse fetal outcomes and heavy drinking is clear in clinical and experimental studies. Because of the shortcomings of research techniques, however, a consensus on the effects of low and moderate concentrations has not been reached. Disagreements can be traced to the problems inherent in relying on personal reports to precisely determine alcohol consumption and to the use of different terms in classifying drinking patterns. Growth retardation, congenital anomalies, neurologic involvement, and spontaneous abortions have been observed clinically only in the heaviest drinking groups, although the terminology used to categorize these groups has varied. Animal experimentation confirms the hypothesis of a dose-response effect with a minimum threshold. Despite the inherent problems of various laboratory techniques, the vast body of experimental data consistently demonstrates that the sustained effects of alcohol occur only when exposure is at least 2 g/kg/per day or BACs are 100 mg percent, no matter what the species or regimen (Randall and Riley, 1981; Fabro, 1982; Randall, 1982). Precise safe levels or thresholds for humans cannot be extrapolated from animal research. The consistency of findings across species, however, clearly indicates that adverse pregnancy outcome is associated with high levels of consumption. There is no empirical evidence of any risk from low levels of consumption.

Assessing risk

The clinician must assess the level of risk for women who have been drinking heavily. Families often request help in deciding whether to continue or terminate a pregnancy. An estimate of the risks within the limits of current knowledge should be made. Case reports provided an early understanding of the problems associated with alcoholism during pregnancy. While cases must be used to identify and describe diseases, they usually represent the most severe form of the problem. Since the milder effects of alcohol and positive outcomes are not reported, overly pessimistic prognoses result. The ability to estimate the incidence or severity of alcohol-related anomalies is limited. Single cases may lead to unwarranted etiological inferences since the role of other factors such as genetics, drug use, chromosomal damage, maternal illness, poor nutrition, and stress cannot be adequately analyzed. Although associations between alcohol and anomalies can be suggested by a single case, causality cannot be confirmed.

The frequency of adverse outcomes in the pregnancies of chronically alcoholic women initially led to recommendations for early termination of pregnancy for women who abuse alcohol (Jones et al, 1974). The sampling methodology used to gather the data which led to this suggestion must be questioned (Rosett, 1974). On the basis of national surveys of drinking practices, one would expect that among 55,000 pregnant women, 2750 (5%) would be heavy drinkers. Jones et al found 23 cases of conspicuous, chronic alcoholism, which probably represented the extremes of the physical, psychological, and sociological ravages of alcoholism. The outlook for children of all heavy drinkers should not be assessed on the basis of the heaviest drinkers in the population. Majewski et al (1978) have stated that therapeutic abortions are indicated for all alcoholics in the chronic stage. For women in the crucial phase, close scrutiny is warranted. In the prodromal stage, they do not believe that abortions are indicated.

Analysis of the incidence of FAS and FAE among heavy drinking women is helpful in estimating the risk for individual patients. Epidemiological studies suggest that between 2% and 10% of the children of alcohol abusers demonstrate FAS. Alcohol related anomalies have been observed in 9 of 70 (13%) infants born to the heaviest drinkers (Hanson et al, 1978). Adverse outcome is associated with advanced stages of maternal alcoholism as reflected in the high morbidity and mortality rate among mothers of FAS children (Majewski, 1981; Véghelyi et al, 1978; Fitze et al, 1978; Clarren, 1982) (see Chapter 5).

In review, the risk of adverse pregnancy outcome is high among chronic alcohol-dependent women. The question remains of which women among alcoholics are at risk and which are not. No simple formula is available for determining the risk for individual women. Physicians and other health care professionals must work with parents to assess risks and benefits individually.

Determining alcohol's effects

Clinicians must also determine the precise nature of the risk which alcohol poses to the fetus. It is clear that maternal alcohol abuse is associated with prenatal and postnatal growth retardation. The relationship between alcohol abuse and either congenital anomalies or mental retardation is less clear. It is sometimes difficult to define what is "abnormal" since the normal range of variability in human development is so great. Only when examiners use standardized criteria and are blind to information about maternal behavior during pregnancy can patterns of anomalies be described consistently and objectively. Bias results from many factors. For example, organ systems are typically not viewed in isolation but are examined as parts of the whole person. Facial characteristics, size, and neurologic status may alert the examiner to look for minor anomalies and perhaps exaggerate their significance, whereas they might otherwise have been viewed as within the range of normal. Furthermore, when the examiner is aware of maternal alcohol consumption, sharper scrutiny may be given to some features. If the drinking history is obtained retrospectively, mothers of abnormal babies may be questioned with greater skepticism than mothers of healthy children.

CONGENITAL MALFORMATIONS

Congenital anomalies reported in case studies are not a strong basis for proving a cause and effect relationship. In case reports, the most minute abnormalities are described, with little discrimination of etiology. The developing fetus is at risk from many variables, particularly when the mother is an alcohol-dependent woman with multiple physiologic and social problems. Case studies cannot delineate the importance of each risk factor. Often, patients are brought to the attention of the investigators because of their apparent malformations, and maternal alcohol dependence is diagnosed subsequently. These children represent a biased sample and cannot be the basis for determining if children of alcoholic mothers have different or more abnormalities than other children.

Malformations cannot be definitively associated with alcohol exposure when they are observed in children who do not meet the minimal diagnostic criteria of FAS. Scheiner et al (1979) described FAS in a child whose mother stopped drinking prior to pregnancy. The diagnosis was disputed with comment on the unfortunate circumstance that single cases with clinically insecure diagnoses can lead to false conclusions (Smith and Graham, 1979). Herrmann et al (1980) reported abnormalities in 11 "FAS" children. While they demonstrated a wide range of abnormalities, they did not consistently conform to the primary diagnostic criteria for FAS (facial features, growth retardation, and CNS effects.) Systematic data on maternal alcohol consumption was not available for every case. Six mothers were positively identified as alcoholic. Heavy drinking was probable for five mothers, two of whom used alcohol as well as several other substances. In another series of 20 cases described as FAS, seven did not demonstrate typical facies (Lipson et al, 1983). Of the remaining 13, growth parameters were unknown in one, and central nervous system assessment was not available in three. Associations described in these reports must be evaluated cautiously.

Prospective studies allow researchers to consistently define standards and assess confounding factors. Bias can be created indirectly by features of the study design. In the prospective studies sponsored by NIAAA, an effort was made for the examiner to be unaware of maternal factors. The Loma Linda, Cleveland, and Boston studies were designed so that all babies born to the defined cohort were examined. An increased incidence of anomalies was observed among the babies of heavy drinkers but no specific pattern could be detected. In the Seattle prospective study, 163 neonates were presented in pairs to the examiner, who knew only that one had been born to a mother in the heaviest drinking category and one was a control infant born the same day to an abstinent or light drinking woman (Hanson et al, 1978). More neonates exposed to alcohol demonstrated a pattern of anomalies similar to FAS. Since one baby in each pair was known to be born to a heavy drinker, an unconscious bias may have influenced the number and nature of anomalies observed in the smaller infants within each pair.

Animal experimentation can circumvent many of the obstacles in clinical research. Rodents are used most commonly and considerable information is available about the normal physiology and social behavior of genetically pure strains bred for research purposes. Short gestation and rapid development allow investigations to be completed quickly with low purchase and maintenance costs. Mice are sensitive to teratogenic effects and demonstrate physiologic abnormalities. Rats are less likely to develop malformations but their learning and activity patterns are appropriate for behavioral research.

The beagle dog is an inbred strain on which there is a large body of physiologic and pharmacologic information. Although beagle dogs will not ingest alcohol voluntarily, they can be trained to accept a gastric tube and swallow administered alcohol without resistance. The pharmacokinetics of ethanol in the beagle is similar to that in humans, so data on dose-effects can be extrapolated to humans. Their ability to sustain pregnancy over a wide range of ethanol doses makes it possible to study the effects of various concentrations of alcohol. Miniature swine are the only species used experimentally that consume alcohol voluntarily over many years. Consequently, studies can be done on the effects of alcohol over several litters farrowed by the same alcoholic dam.

Monkeys are closest to humans in their placental structure, which differs from that of rodents and dogs. They have single births rather than litters and they have an extended period of development in utero beyond the embryonic stage. Homogeneous genetic structure has been inbred in rodents but is not found in primates. Some subhuman primate behaviors, such as infant–mother relationships and lengthy periods of socialization, are similar to those in humans. However, monkeys are extremely costly to purchase and maintain, and they rarely voluntarily drink large quantities of ethanol. Intravenous administration of ethanol often interferes with conception. Monkeys which have been conditioned to drink alcohol often stop spontaneously when they become pregnant.

Differences between species limit extrapolation of animal data on anomalies. Alcohol's effects are mediated by genetic susceptibilities, pharmacodynamics, and by physiologic differences in placental structure. Chernoff (1977) reported significant differences between strains of a single species: alcohol's effects were more pronounced in CBA mice than in other mouse strains given equivalent doses. Differences were thought to be related to the genetic capacity to metabolize alcohol. Sulik et al (1981) produced cranio-facial dysmorphology similar to FAS in C57 mice exposed to ethanol. However, similar dysmorphology occurred in 12% of the controls, suggesting genetic predisposition to facial anomalies.

Experimental research clearly demonstrates that alcohol has the capacity to affect the developing fetus in all species in diverse ways. Just as in the adult, multiple organ systems are susceptible to the effects of excessive alcohol. Exposure of embryos to specific doses at specific stages has demonstrated that the nature and severity of anomalies are dependent on dose and timing. The lack of a specific pattern reflects alcohol's multiple effects on fetal development and does not call into question its teratogenic power.

MENTAL RETARDATION

Mental retardation is often cited as the most devastating effect of in utero exposure to alcohol. Children of alcohol-dependent women often show impaired intellectual functioning and other psychological handicaps. Few prospective studies have investigated the effects of various drinking patterns or have traced the development of alcohol-exposed children. Most evaluations of the effects of in utero alcohol exposure on behavior have been based on clinical observations or case series. In one series, several different tests were performed with children ranging in age from 9 months to 21 years (Streissguth et al, 1981). The consistency of the observed psychological handicaps may reflect the severity with which the children were affected. FAS children who are not severely dysmorphic show higher IQs, better social adaptation, and improvement over time (Seidenberg and Majewski, 1978; Steinhausen et al, 1982). An association between moderate alcohol use and developmental decrements has been observed by only one group of researchers (Streissguth et al, 1980). This result has been criticized because children of women reporting ingesting a very wide range of alcohol (from 1 to 4 oz) were analyzed as one group (Fabro, 1982).

The in utero effects of alcohol become more difficult to identify as each developmental year passes. Dynamic interactions between the infant and mother are altered by the effects of alcohol abuse on the infant and on maternal behavior. The complex interrelationships of environmental stress, inadequate parenting, lack of enrichment, poor nutrition, and other associated risk factors limit clinical studies. One study reported no associations between maternal drinking before or during pregnancy and the quality of environmental stimulation (Ragozin et al, 1978). Among the 51 women who participated, none were heavy drinkers. Unfortunately data was not obtained on the mothers' alcohol consumption after the birth of the child because the authors felt that questions about current habits might jeopardize the women's future participation in the study. This reluctance reflects a bias on the part of the researchers that might affect interpretation as well as collection of data. We do not agree that questions about alcohol use alienate participants. In our experience, women were not offended when questions were asked honestly and sincerely. Omission of essential information prevents resolution of the crucial question of the relative importance of in utero exposure and environmental deprivation in developmental problems.

Although the association between socioeconomic status (SES) and scores on tests of intelligence is well established, most reports of development in FAS cases have not described SES. A review of 38 cases in the English language literature revealed that developmental scores were significantly higher for middle-class FAS children than for those from families of lower SES (Casey, 1983).

Long-term developmental studies are needed to determine the persistent effects of various levels of alcohol consumption and to control for confounding factors which could themselves account for mental deficiency (Neugut, 1982). Because of the complexity in the clinical situation, data from experimental research must be utilized.

Experimental studies clearly demonstrate a relationship between in utero exposure to high doses of alcohol and hyperactivity. Reports on alcohol's effects on learning patterns are contradictory. Methodologic issues pertaining to both mother and pup may explain some of the differences. In the rat and mouse, postnatal maternal behavior and lactation can affect development, independent of prenatal factors. Cross-fostering of prenatally exposed offspring to surrogate mothers eliminates the problems caused by changes in maternal behavior, but it introduces new problems by interfering with normal mother–infant interactions. Handling of newborn pups can cause the mother to reject the pups with later behavioral sequelae.

Results may vary according to the dose administered. In some instances, doses may be too low. When Riley et al (1979b) tested reversal learning in rat pups whose mothers were fed liquid alcohol, teratogenicity was not observed among the group in which 17% of calories was derived from alcohol but was observed in the group receiving 35% of calories as alcohol. Bond (1981) reviewed the experimental data and suggested that intellectual impairment results when fetuses are exposed to at least 6–7 g/kg per day. Concentrations of administered doses of alcohol can be excessive. Mukherjee and Hodgen (1982) observed a collapse of the umbilical vasculature following injection of a bolus of alcohol equivalent to 530 ml of 80 proof whiskey (Kimball, 1983). Administration of this dose in this form is in no way analogous to the use of beverage alcohol. Before any hypothesis is accepted or rejected, it should be tested at multiple doses which all have clinical relevance.

The age at which animals are tested may also influence results. Experiments which sacrifice pups seven days after exposure to high doses of alcohol demonstrate impaired development (Sulik et al, 1981). However, restitution in cell development can occur in utero (Anders and Persaud, 1980; Dreosti et al, 1981; O'Shea and Kaufman, 1981). Early differences in the Purkinje cells of the rat brain were not observed later in gestation (Volk et al, 1981). Behaviors have changed over time, suggesting developmental delays rather than intellectual impairment. Early deficits in response inhibition diminished with maturity (Riley et al, 1979a; Riley et al, 1979b). Bond (1981) concluded that young animals' performance (< 70 days) was impeded by hyperactivity which lessened with time. Differences observed in learning patterns in adult rats (> 90 days) reflected impairment. Experimental cohorts should be evaluated at several gestational and developmental stages to evaluate the permanent or transitory nature of alcohol's effects.

The type of tests used and the different behavioral capabilities of animal species also affect conclusions. Most research protocols test the highest level of behavior of which each species is capable. Since performance may be less impaired in simple than in complex tasks, deficiencies or delays may not be demonstrated in species not capable of complex behavioral tasks. Insult to particular brain regions may cause specific behavioral aberrations which may not be apparent in all test modes. Multiple and varied tests over a long span of time are required for a full understanding.

In conclusion, when methodologic issues are considered, consistent findings on alcohol's effects emerge. Although there are unresolved areas, it is clear that the children of alcohol-dependent women are at risk for a variety of physiologic and developmental problems, the nature of which cannot easily be specified. Growth retardation is the most clearly manifested. There is also an increased incidence of nonspecific abnormalities affecting multiple organ systems. Impaired learning and abnormal behavioral patterns occur with higher frequency. The potential for remediation should be further explored and specific techniques tested and developed.

Differentiating alcohol's effects

Despite the cumulative experimental evidence, some question whether the adverse effects result from heavy alcohol consumption or from the overall lifestyle of the alcoholic. In every prospective study, heavy drinking was associated with other risk factors that have been independently linked with poor pregnancy outcome, including smoking, use of other drugs, stress, and malnutrition. Any statistical analysis of alcohol's effects should consider the role of these other possible causal factors. Investigators should use methods which can analyze rare events since both the pattern of alcohol consumption and the rate of anomalies are highly skewed. Heavy alcohol use occurs among a small group of pregnant women who consume far greater amounts of alcohol than the rest of the population (USDHHS, 1981). Similarly, growth retardation and abnormalities are uncommon occurrences in the total population.

Most studies have utilized multiple regression and canonical correlation techniques which evaluate the unique contribution of multiple independent variables and provide summary information about differences in group means. However, as in all statistical techniques, it is not possible to control for every variable. In addition, variables which are included in the analysis are all given equal status, regardless of their clinical or biologic importance. These techniques were not designed to describe individuals or subgroups. Large numbers of people within categories are required to demonstrate associations. Since normal distributions are assumed, data on atypical individuals undergoes transformations to bring it closer to the norm. When alcohol use is viewed on an interval scale, the impact of frequent moderate doses is impossible to differentiate from occasional high levels. Further, the J-shaped distribution curve for alcohol consumption is revised to a linear curve with a constant slope. Threshold phenomena cannot be distinguished from linear effects.

Conclusions from many prospective studies have been based on variations from a mean, and the percent of variance explained by the independent variables as derived from multiple regressions analyses. Cohen and Cohen (1975) suggest that reports of decrements from the mean are not sufficient. The impact of one variable upon another can best be understood by knowing the percent of variance explained. The small amount of variance accounted for raises questions about the clinical significance of the findings. In

Streissguth et al's (1980) study of motor and mental development at 8 months, all variables measured accounted for 6% of the total variance in infant performance; alcohol use explained approximately 1–2%. Kuzma and Sokol (1982) examined 44 potential determinants and found 11 to have statistical significance with birthweight. The three most important determinants (duration of gestation, mother's pre-pregnancy weight, and weight gain) explained 29% of the variance; the other eight accounted for an additional 1.2%. Hingson et al (1982) reported that 8 of 22 variables tested were found to have independent associations with birthweight ($p < 0.01$). Gestational age accounted for 29% of the variance; seven additional variables explained 12.1%. Harlap and Shiono (1980) analyzed the incidence of second trimester spontaneous abortions. Alcohol, cigarettes, ethnicity, age, parity, previous induced and spontaneous abortions together accounted for less than 1% of the spontaneous abortion rate (personal communication).

The amount of variance explained by each independent variable may be influenced by the number of cases in the subgroups (Cohen and Cohen, 1975). The null hypothesis may be falsely accepted in samples with small subgroups. Kuzma and Sokol (1982) have demonstrated that alcohol's effect on birthweight occurred only among the 3% of gravidas drinking most frequently. One would not expect that this group could contribute greatly to the variance. The analysis of small subgroups is further complicated by the loss of cases with missing information. In the study by Kuzma and Sokol (1982), 4% were excluded from analysis. The sample of Hingson et al (1982) was reduced by 21%. The excluded group differed significantly from the group included on several variables: more alcohol use before and during pregnancy, more cigarette smokers, and more medical illnesses.

Data analysis is a craft which employs statistical techniques to make data yield its meaning. Some data is not appropriate for traditional analytical methods. Scientific and mathematical judgment must be used to provide new ways to analyze complex situations. Marcus and Hans (1982) have suggested that Guttman's Multidimensional Scalogram Analysis (MSA) is relevant for the study of the effects of toxins on child development. In this technique, a mapping sentence organizes the universe of observation and looks at the structure of individuals' profiles. It allows relationships among variables and subjects to be examined, yet retains the original form of the items. There are no assumptions that the data have interval or ordinal properties. Profiles of individuals can be identified and comparisons can be made between multiple subgroups and controls. However, no statistical techniques are currently available to evaluate the findings.

In our study at Boston City Hospital, we attempted to overcome the problems of studying events that occur rarely by using a matched-pairs technique (Rosett et al, 1983b). Each woman who continued to drink heavily or who reduced mid-pregnancy was matched to every moderate and rare drinker who was similar to her on eight variables thought to influence fetal development. This technique facilitated analyzing the impact of alcohol and other risk factors on neonatal outcome within subsets of drinking groups. Sustained heavy drinking was associated with adverse fetal development. The association existed despite the presence or absence of other risk factors. No other relationships were observed between drinking patterns and neonatal status. Matched-pair techniques have been used by others to study a small number of women reporting particular habit patterns, such as marijuana and other drug use, and birth outcome (Whiting et al, 1978; Fried, 1982; Greenland et al, 1982).

Summary

Research on alcohol's effects on fetal development has become more sophisticated in the past few years. The recognition of methodological limitations has influenced recent analysis of data and has stimulated scientists to formulate techniques to overcome some of the problems. Some issues, including the extrapolation of dose-response from animal data to humans, will never be resolved. Although one can draw conclusions about safe levels of alcohol consumption from clinical and experimental research, there will never be definitive answers or absolute safety. Questions will always arise about dose, timing, species sensitivity, type of test, and statistical techniques. Some will use this uncertainty to justify prohibiting all alcohol use during pregnancy. Others will consider that threshold effects occur with most teratogens and have been observed in animals experimentally exposed to ethanol. Hypothesizing that thresholds to alcohol must also occur in humans, they will urge caution during pregnancy without overstating the danger.

Eight

Therapy

There is an overwhelming body of evidence that heavy drinking adversely affects fetal growth and development. Identifying and treating problem drinking before and during pregnancy is an effective prevention strategy. Experimental evidence suggests that alcohol can interfere not only with organogenesis but with growth and development throughout gestation. Reducing heavy alcohol consumption in mid-pregnancy will modify some of the adverse biochemical and physiologic effects; although structural malformations may persist, early delays in growth and development can show restitution.

During pregnancy most women are concerned about the changes in their own bodies and the well-being of the child they will bear. Strong feelings of responsibility motivate them to adopt health habits that are beneficial to the fetus. At this time, they are receptive to therapy focused on reduction of drinking.

Identification of drinking patterns

Society's ambivalence toward women who drink interferes with the physician's ability to diagnose alcohol abuse in the pregnant woman and the patient's ability to ask for help. Because of mixed feelings about alcohol use some physicians are reluctant to ask about drinking patterns. They project their own moralistic attitudes onto women

who drink, and imagine that patients will be offended if they inquire. The physician's embarrassment and defensiveness prevents
the patient from accurately reporting her drinking behavior. Problem drinkers both seek and fear medical intervention and rely on
the doctor to aggressively pursue the diagnosis. They often will not
request help directly, but are prepared to discuss drinking with their
physicians and will not immediately reject treatment (Jones and
Helrich, 1972; Murphy, 1980).

Alcohol abuse occurs among obstetric and gynecologic patients
more often than health care providers suspect. Sokol et al (1980)
reported that a prenatal screening program identified 11% of the
population as problem drinkers, whereas nonsystematic identification had only shown 1.9%. Similarly, Larsson (1983) reported that
11% of the study population was found to be drinking heavily although none had previously been identified. Systematically including
a drinking history in every initial evaluation is the most practical
way to identify problem drinking. Pregnant women usually do not
fit the stereotype of the alcoholic since they are young and in the
early stages of the disease. Although women who drink heavily
differ statistically from other pregnant women on a series of behavioral and demographic traits, these traits have low predictive power
and are ineffective as specific clinical markers (Weiner et al, 1983).

At Boston City Hospital, we developed a brief Ten Question
Drinking History, adapted from a long questionnaire used in our
research protocol. This was incorporated into the prenatal clinic
record to be administered routinely as part of the initial examination
(see Appendix) (Rosett et al, 1981). Separate direct inquiry is made
about the frequency, quantity, and variability of the consumption
of beer, wine, and liquor since the validity of self-reports improves
when specific questions are asked about the use of each beverage
(Cahalan et al, 1969). The first nine questions ascertain present
drinking patterns. Inquiry is made in a fashion which assumes alcohol use and thereby diminishes moral projections. The tenth question explores changes in drinking habits during the past year. This
is important because it allows for discussion of previous drinking
patterns which often provides a point of departure for validating
reports of current use.

When the ten questions are asked in a direct, nonjudgmental
fashion, most patients accept the clinician's concern and respond
honestly. Simple introductory statements reassure the patient that

the questions are being asked in an effort to improve patient care. Patients who answer evasively should calmly and firmly be engaged in further discussion. Defensive reactions to the questions often indicate alcohol problems.

When the Ten Question Drinking History was incorporated in the prenatal intake in a context similar to that used to obtain information on nutrition, smoking, and other medical data, it proved to be reliable (Weiner et al, 1982). Drinking patterns reported to the clinic staff were consistent with those obtained by research interviewers. The reliability of the questionnaire was further tested by Larsson (1983), who reported good agreement between two occasions of history taking (range 89–100%). Answering the ten questions required less than five minutes when women did not report a drinking problem. For women who were abusing alcohol, the questionnaire provided a basis for discussing the possible adverse effects of their drinking and for initiating supportive counselling.

To assess drinking patterns, data on consumption of beer, wine, and liquor were combined. Weekly rates were converted to monthly rates, and quantities were standardized so that a "drink" was the amount of beverage containing 0.5 oz AA. Women who reported at least 45 drinks a month with five or more on some occasions were considered heavy drinkers. Many different drinking patterns, varying in both frequency and quantity of drinking, were reported by the women who met the criteria for heavy drinking. Frequency of drinking ranged from daily to 1–2 times a week. Variability was observed within the group as well as in individual drinking patterns.

The particular format for inquiring about alcohol use should fit the style of the professional. Sokol and Miller (1980) suggest that reliable drinking histories can be obtained more easily if alcohol use among family members has been discussed as part of the family history. This paves the way for further inquiry by underscoring the fact that alcohol use is of medical importance and concern to the physician. Questions about the patient's own alcohol use are asked following questions about cigarette use. In the context of personal habits, patients are not offended when asked "Do you ever drink any wine, beer, or mixed drinks?" When patients reply that they do not drink, no further questions are asked. Most patients respond that they sometimes have a drink. Query is first made about past drinking behavior since separating it from present behavior avoids unnecessary resistance. Questions about current behavior are asked next. A range of expected responses of relatively high amounts is suggested, for example, "One or two six-packs at a time?". Women who do not abuse alcohol will not be offended by this line of questioning. Women who drink heavily will usually respond positively. When heavy drinking is indicated, information is gathered on the circumstances as well as the amount and pattern of use.

Other protocols for obtaining information on alcohol abuse have been designed for use by health care professionals with a variety of patients and can be used with the prenatal patient. The Michigan Alcoholism Screening Test (MAST) consists of 25 questions which focus on psychosocial disruption related to drinking (Selzer, 1971) (see Appendix). It is usually presented as a self-administered test. Although it does not quantify the amount of alcohol consumed, it can identify pregnant women with drinking problems (Sokol et al, 1981). A ten page self-administered questionnaire (SAQ) has been proven reliable with obstetric and gynecologic patients (Russell, 1982). When used in conjunction with a questionnaire administered by the physician and a medical record review, sensitivity was 90%. About 20 minutes is required to administer the MAST, the SAQ, and most other standardized alcohol surveys. CAGE is a brief questionnaire, consisting of four questions designed to detect alcohol problems (Mayfield et al, 1974) (see Appendix). It is effective for heavy drinkers but does not differentiate other drinking patterns.

Some questions about alcohol use should be avoided. It is preferable not to ask "Do you drink?" since it connotes problem drinking and usually will evoke a negative response. Also, "You don't drink do you?" suggests the socially acceptable reply and will yield little information. When patients sense the professional's discomfort and desire to avoid knowing about alcohol problems they become reluctant to speak candidly. The question "Do you drink socially?" is ineffective because the term "social drinking" has diverse meanings in different social circles.

A careful drinking history obtained in the context of helping the mother to have a healthier child is the most effective technique for ascertaining drinking patterns. Objective means of measuring alcohol consumption are not yet available for clinical use (see Chapter 7). Heavy drinking pregnant women place their fetus at risk before they themselves show classic physical and biochemical signs of alcoholism.

Treatment strategies

Treatment of heavy drinking during pregnancy should be directed toward attaining and sustaining abstinence as quickly as possible. Therapeutic outcome is affected by the attitudes of the health professional. The expectation of success improves counselling results (Chappell and Schnoll, 1977). One obstacle to recovery is the patient's despair over her inability to stop drinking and her remorse for the damage she may have done to the fetus. When health care providers share this hopelessness, patients feel unable to master the problem. The professional's sincere concern and efforts directed toward the positive outcome of pregnancy help motivate the patient to abstain. Women will respond more positively to a hopeful message of the potential benefits of reduction than to a pessimistic prognosis of fetal damage. Provocation of guilt and increased self-denigration is intolerable to many women and may lead them to increase their alcohol consumption during pregnancy. Information conveyed in a supportive manner rather than a critical and negative manner is more conducive to behavioral change. The two approaches are illustrated below:

Negative approach	Positive approach
Warn of serious hazards.	Emphasize woman's ability to reduce risk.
Reprimand about responsibility to fetus.	Support maternal desires.
Castigate for being a bad mother.	Promote confidence in potential to be a good mother.
Emphasize complications of intoxication.	Discuss benefits of sobriety.

Drinking patterns change throughout life and particularly during the early stages of pregnancy. At Boston City Hospital, a number of rare and moderate drinkers reported an aversion to alcohol with the onset of pregnancy. Among the women who were drinking heavily at the time of registration, 60% reported that their level of drinking was lower than at other times in their lives. Concern for the baby was cited most often as the reason for changing drinking habits. Few heavy drinking women reported a change in taste for alcohol. Marked reduction among heavy drinkers has been reported in several other studies of pregnant women (Little et al, 1976; Fried et al, 1980; Kline et al, 1980; Kuzma and Kissinger, 1981; Sokol et al, 1981; Minor and Van Dort, 1982). With the exception of the Cleveland program (Sokol et al, 1981), counselling was not provided in any of these programs which were designed to investigate drinking patterns but not to provide therapy. The spontaneous changes in drinking patterns suggest that pregnancy is an optimum time for therapy focused on reducing alcohol use.

Counselling for heavy drinkers should be initiated as soon as alcohol abuse is identified. Since alcohol has the capacity to adversely affect each stage of fetal development, the earlier in pregnancy that heavy drinking ceases, the greater is the potential for an improved outcome. Therapy should begin with the primary care provider and should not be postponed until a specialist is available. Most of the women are young and in the early stages of alcohol abuse. They do not view themselves as alcoholics and will respond to therapy integrated with routine care more readily than to referral to alcohol specialists. Advice to give to women with moderate and light drinking patterns is discussed in Chapter 9.

Treatment experience at Boston City Hospital

At Boston City Hospital, all women identified as heavy drinkers were advised that they would have a better chance of having a healthy baby if they stopped drinking (Rosett et al, 1983a). They were invited to participate in counselling sessions that were conducted in the prenatal clinic, and scheduled to coincide with routine obstetrical appointments. The first session, with the project psychiatrist, included a diagnostic interview and an independent drinking history. Evaluation of treatment needs began with an assessment of the woman's strengths, including her style of coping with anxiety and depression, her capacity to sustain close relationships with others, and her resourcefulness in times of adversity. A specific and detailed history of her patterns of substance abuse had therapeutic and prognostic importance; a past history of successful withdrawal followed by a sustained drug-free period is a positive indicator.

Followup sessions with the project psychiatrist and/or counsellor averaged one half-hour. The frequency of sessions ranged from one to four times a month. The schedule usually was determined by the woman's obstetrical needs; however, when more frequent counselling was indicated, additional appointments were made. Women who needed supportive therapy more often than once a week were referred to specialized centers.

An interim history of alcohol consumption was included in each session with a discussion both of quantity consumed and circumstances surrounding use. The alcoholic content of "drinks" of beer, wine, and whiskey were defined. Women were advised that substitution of one beverage for another did not constitute reduction. Myths that beer or wine were not as harmful as whiskey were dispelled. Abstinence was praised. When a woman reported that she had continued or resumed drinking, she was again told of the potential benefits of reduction. The following kinds of statements seemed most helpful: "You have a better chance of having a healthy baby if you stop drinking" or "I am concerned about your drinking and would like to help you." Criticism and provocation of guilt were avoided since the general experience in alcoholism treatment has been that guilt and fear increase alcohol abuse.

One of the critical goals of treatment is to build self-esteem, commonly lacking in alcoholics. Many women put pressure on themselves to be "perfect" mothers, based on expectations developed throughout life. When ideals and reality differ, feelings of depression and self-hate develop. This is particularly true for problem drinking women who internalize society's view that drinking while mothering is bad. In this frame of mind, women accept responsibility for all problems and feel guilty for "wrongs" they have done to the fetus. They need help to recognize that they have not behaved willfully and maliciously. They also need support from health professionals in the form of a hopeful message that by abstaining for the remainder of the pregnancy they are able to improve their chances of having a healthy baby. Most women experience a spectrum of emotions in anticipation of childbirth, ranging from love and joy to apprehension and fear of impending pain and inadequacy. These complex feelings can overwhelm a woman who is guilt-ridden because of her drinking. Open discussion of this ambivalence can minimize the guilt and depression.

Frequently, prenatal episodes of heavy drinking are associated with ambivalence toward the pregnancy. The woman's attitudes and those of her spouse should be explored to determine whether they want to have the baby, and areas of conflict should be identified. Heavy drinking may be a manifestation of marital discord or a couple's doubts about whether they want to maintain their relationship. There may be fear on the woman's part that a man other than the husband is the father of the baby. Women sometimes experience guilt related to sexual behavior years earlier. Even sophisticated women may believe that adolescent activity such as masturbation or premarital sex will be punished through a deformed child. Other knowledgeable women are concerned about the mechanisms of childbirth and become obsessed about how the baby emerges from their body, even if they have already delivered a baby. Such obsessional ideas can sometimes be relieved by a supportive discussion with the obstetrician. However, at other times they may be manifestations of more severe emotional illness. If obsessions and excessive drinking do not cease within two weeks, referral to a psychiatrist or a mental health facility is indicated.

While counselling at Boston City Hospital focused on reducing alcohol use, other issues important to each woman and to the positive outcome of her pregnancy were considered. Help with real life situations was provided by practical suggestions and referrals to appropriate hospital departments and community agencies. Diet, smoking, and use of other drugs were discussed. Many women were confused about their own anatomy and details of the birth process. Fears of delivery were alleviated through an educational approach. A diagram of placental circulation helped explain alcohol's ability to cross the placenta and alter fetal growth and development. Birth control methods were reviewed. Although this information had been presented in childbirth classes conducted by the regular clinic staff, our patients needed supplementary individualized discussion.

The heavy-drinking women frequently were concerned about the possibility of having permanently damaged their fetus. An estimate of the risks of heavy drinking within the limitations of current knowledge was presented to the patient. The possibility of reducing risks by abstaining for the remainder of the pregnancy was presented positively. Decisions about continuing or terminating the pregnancy depend on the balance between the woman's capacity to abstain from alcohol and her wish to become a parent, as well as on individual philosophic and religious beliefs. No simple formula is available.

The woman's relationships with her family, and particularly with the father of the baby, were explored. Help was enlisted from family members who could provide support. The negative influence of some family members was acknowledged. Women who drink heavily often associate with men who also drink heavily and they reinforce each other's drinking behavior. Some family members resist getting involved in treatment since the woman's new-found sobriety forces changes in family roles and can be threatening. Involvement of family members should be considered whenever possible, even if resistance exists, as it has been observed to be consistently beneficial (Finkelstein et al, 1981).

Women who had developed a physiologic tolerance to alcohol and were drinking over a pint a day were advised to gradually reduce consumption over several days to achieve abstinence. Initial experience with withdrawal of two women who had been drinking more than a quart a day and were hospitalized demonstrated no adverse effects on mother or fetus when alcohol dose was reduced over four days. Outpatient withdrawal of subsequent patients was also without observed complications. Benzodiazepines and other sedative drugs were avoided to minimize teratogenic risks.

In extreme cases, in-patient care may be required to ensure sobriety. One woman was admitted in the 30th week of pregnancy with a BAC of 460 mg percent. She had not attained sobriety by attending Alcoholics Anonymous, mental health centers, and alcohol treatment centers. She had been detoxified four times during her pregnancy. B-scans revealed that fetal weight was in the 3rd percentile at 28 and 34 weeks. At delivery, gestational age was 41 weeks and weight was between the 10th and 25th percentiles. A thin upper lip and flattened philtrum were evident.

Most women were strongly motivated by maternal concerns and did not require the coercive effect of disulfiram (Antabuse), which has been implicated as a potential teratogen. Tissot-Favre and Delatour's (1965) prospective study of five pregnancies with daily maternal exposure to 250–500 mg of disulfiram demonstrated one spontaneous abortion in the second month, two infants born with club feet, and two normal children. Nora et al (1977) conducted a teratogen surveillance program based on a review of 1320 case histories of pregnant women and identified only two in which the infants had been exposed to disulfiram during the first trimester. Both infants had severe limb-reduction anomalies; one had multiple anomalies, including radial aplasia, vertebral fusion and tracheoesophageal fistula, and the other had phocomelia of the legs. They were not known to have been exposed to aclohol or any other established teratogen. Disulfiram inhibits several enzymes, in addition to aldehyde dehydrogenase. One is dopamine beta hydroxylase, which catalyzes the conversion of dopamine to norepinephrine and thus has multiple neurophysiologic functions (Truitt and Walsh, 1971). In addition, the three major metabolites of disulfiram (carbon disulfide, diethylamine, and diethyldithiocarbamate) have been found to be neurotoxic (Rainey, 1977).

Two-thirds of the women who participated in three or more counselling sessions at Boston City Hospital stopped drinking heavily. Information on demographic and behavioral traits gathered in the screening interview did not readily distinguish heavy drinkers who would reduce alcohol consumption from those who would not. Within the two groups, there was a wide range of individual differences in personality, psychopathology, and patterns of alcohol use. Frequency and quantity of alcohol consumption was not a predictor of therapeutic success. Young nulliparous women were more likely to reduce consumption. Women who reported on the survey that they found drinking helpful when nervous or depressed had a less favorable prognosis.

Response to treatment varied. Most women responded relatively quickly and reduced consumption within two weeks. Some were able to stop drinking only when they found alternatives to help them stay sober, which were as diverse as the individuals themselves. Many women reported that they had to change friends in order to eliminate peer pressure to drink. Some actually moved for the duration of the pregnancy to avoid familiar drinking environments or to be with abstinent relatives. Several women who were seen at prenatal registration at Boston City Hospital and subsequently obtained prenatal care at a neighborhood health center reported that they stopped drinking heavily on the basis of the brief advice which followed the survey interview. They appreciated the interest and concern of the counsellor and took seriously the recommendation that they would have a better chance for a healthier child if they abstained. This message, individually delivered by a professional interested in their health habits, was a powerful motivating force.

Phases of problem drinking

A three-phase classification of problem drinking was useful in designing treatment strategies. Classification was based on motivating factors rather than on quantity or duration of use. The phases are not necessarily progressive although some women had moved from one to the next.

SOCIAL PROBLEM DRINKING

Women in this phase drank because of social pressures. Consumption of alcohol was an essential ingredient in their marriages and friendships as well as in the social lives of their communities. When they tried to abstain several experienced pressure from friends and relatives to continue to drink. Feeling lonely and bored, some used alcohol to gain the illusion of rapid passage of time. Many women in this phase were able to stop drinking for the duration of pregnancy on the basis of brief supportive counselling with information that they had a better chance of having a healthy child if they abstained. Concern from the father of the baby or other family members also was a powerful motivating factor. In the absence of this encouragement, some women moved to live with nondrinking relatives. Many had to develop alternative social and recreational activities. For women in the social phase, support and referral to appropriate agencies and self-help groups were most important.

Case A

Sheila, a 20-year-old primipara, was unmarried and living with her mother when she registered for prenatal care in her third month. She had left school at the end of the ninth grade and soon after began drinking daily. She and her mother shared a six pack of beer and either a pint of fortified wine or a half-pint of vodka during a three-hour period. The father of the baby, whom she saw regularly, drank about a half pint of vodka daily. During the five years preceding the pregnancy she had several hospital admissions for lacerations associated with intoxication. She smoked about half a pack of cigarettes a day and occasionally used marijuana. Her poor diet improved as a result of nutritional counselling but it remained marginal. Information about the effects of alcohol on pregnancy motivated some periods of abstinence. At other times she drank occasional beers and binged. We continued to praise her attempts at abstinence and avoided criticism or guilt provocation. In the third trimester, following a death in the family, she spent six weeks with her grandmother who allowed no alcohol in the house. During this time, she attained total abstinence which she maintained until delivery. Her son weighed 3232 grams, average for gestational age. He was normal on examination with some minor anomalies of the lips and philtrum characteristic of FAS.

SYMPTOM PROBLEM DRINKING

In this phase, women used drinking to relieve a range of psychological symptoms and were dependent on alcohol to alter mood and perception. Some sought relief from depression associated with family disruption and parental loss. Others, feeling helpless and overwhelmed by environmental pressures, used alcohol to blur their awareness of fear, confusion, and discouragement. For many, pregnancy exacerbated stressful situations in their lives. The added physical and social responsibilities caused ambivalent feelings towards motherhood. These women were particularly sensitive to the attitudes others had towards them and often misinterpreted comments from staff members. Realistic discussion of conflicts about their roles as mothers helped to reduce feelings of inadequacy. They needed repetition of information about pregnancy and the birth process which had been presented by other staff members. Women in this group required extensive counselling and support with a variety of social problems as well as with the normal crises secondary to pregnancy.

Case B

Deborah, a 19-year-old primipara who lived with her mother, drank rarely prior to pregnancy. During the third month, she and a girlfriend began drinking every night until they became intoxicated. She had no contact with the father of the baby. Because of her mother's objections, she did not have an abortion. Her mother also restricted physical activities that she deemed dangerous to the baby, advising her not to exercise, play ball, or lift her arms above her head. Friends were also reluctant to have her join their athletic activities. The mother encouraged alcohol consumption to relieve anxieties, a remedy she herself used. We provided Deborah with detailed information about pregnancy, nutrition, and the birth process, all of which concerned her greatly. Her older brother provided alternative activities to replace athletics. She quickly achieved sobriety. She delivered a baby weighing 3119 grams, normal on newborn examination. Since she had no support at home and was overwhelmed by the impending responsibilities of motherhood, referral was made to the infant development unit to improve parenting skills.

ALCOHOL DEPENDENCE (ALCOHOLISM)

Women in this phase had developed a physiologic tolerance and a dependency on alcohol and met DSM III criteria for the diagnosis of alcoholism. Most were consuming between a pint and a quart of liquor a day or its equivalent. Several had developed medical complications secondary to alcohol use, including hepatitis, pancreatitis, and nondiabetic ketoacidosis. In addition to their medical needs, they required extensive assistance with child care and social service problems. In two cases abstinence was achieved following a court decree that child custody was contingent upon successful treatment. Alcoholism treatment centers, halfway houses, and Alcoholics Anonymous groups provided supplementary therapy and support.

Case C

Brenda was 27 years old and in the 6th month of her pregnancy when admitted to the Boston City Hospital Obstetrical Service for severe abdominal pain. Two previous pregnancies had terminated with spontaneous abortions. She reported that she had begun drinking wine when she was 12 years old. For the past 11 years, she had been regularly drinking to intoxication, estimating that she consumed more than two quarts of vodka as well as 12 cans of beer a day. When she felt ill, she refrained from alcohol for a few days. She did not believe that she had been sober for more than a week during the previous year. She had been in several treatment programs and had been detoxified at least twice prior to this pregnancy. Brenda lived alone, with regular visits from the father of the baby. Her mother also was alcoholic.

During our first meeting, she was annoyed by our intrusion and expressed no motivation to stop drinking nor concern that it might harm the baby. She did not return for prenatal care. Six weeks later she was again admitted for gastritis secondary to alcohol abuse. She reported sobriety following the first hospitalization until a two-day binge caused a recurrence of the gastritis and convinced her of the need for abstinence. Brenda's impulsivity was obvious from scars of wounds self-inflicted while drunk or incurred during violent fights with her mother and other bar patrons.

Before she knew she was pregnant she had used valium, sleeping pills, and two bags of heroin daily. She also reported smoking four packs of cigarettes and drinking 15 cups of coffee daily. She stopped all other drug use early in pregnancy and stopped drinking alcohol for the third trimester. A girl was born at term weighing 2495 grams. Neonatal examination was normal.

Although she had been motivated by the pregnancy to be drug-free, there were doubts about her ability to sustain herself. A court order allowed her custody of the baby with the provision that she attend an alcohol treatment program and that public health nurses visit weekly. Brenda resumed alcoholic drinking when the baby was four months old and lost child custody. With support from the alcoholism clinic, drinking abated and the child was returned to her nine months later.

Referrals

Some women required more intensive therapy than was practical to integrate with routine prenatal care. When women failed to respond within two weeks, referrals were made to specialized alcohol treatment centers. Women who had previous success with Alcoholics Anonymous (AA) or other community groups were encouraged to re-establish these relationships. Some who had relied on their extended families and friends were urged to try the Boston City Hospital Alcoholism Clinic, AA, or church groups. In a few instances, referrals to halfway houses were indicated. Most primary care providers have the skills needed to initiate supportive therapy. While they can be effective with the majority of the problem drinking women, they can not help everyone and should not react with frustration when cures elude them. The availability of consultation and referral sources make primary providers more willing to undertake therapy of heavy drinking. The fear of being "stuck" with a difficult problem has been cited by some health care professionals as their reason for avoiding the initial evaluation and counselling role.

Referrals can be made to psychiatrists and psychologists as well as to clinics and private alcohol treatment centers. Lists of treatment facilities are generally available from the state and community departments of public health. Recovered alcoholics who are in the patient population are a valuable source of information on treatment facilities and support groups. In most areas, there are several AA groups, each of which may appeal to different clients. When making referrals to AA, it is useful to telephone a central AA office and inquire about the compatibility of the several groups for the pregnant woman or new mother.

Alcoholic patients rarely respond to vague referrals. It is crucial to refer them to specific programs and to help arrange the initial appointment. Personal introductions to social workers or alcoholism counsellors on the hospital staff facilitates referrals. AA referral centers will often assign a volunteer member to familiarize women with the program in their community. Following referrals, it is important to maintain discussions with the women about their drinking patterns. They welcome the continued concern, which can be an additional motivating force. If treatment at an alcohol center is not accepted, continued discussion with the primary provider keeps opportunities for therapy open. Even among patients who initially react angrily and overtly reject assistance, information about the benefits of reduction and sustained interest may have beneficial results.

Patients who fail to maintain total abstinence and slip back into alcohol use should be encouraged to try to abstain one day at a time. Supportive reinforcement of success should be emphasized. Punitive invocation of guilt and anxiety make future sobriety more difficult. The social, physical, and psychological components of addiction make complete cessation a difficult task. Treatment must be considered from a long-term perspective.

Intervention with the pregnant problem drinker should be used to establish a relationship which facilitates continuing care for both the mother and the newborn infant. To sustain the gains made in dealing with alcohol abuse during pregnancy, referrals for post-

partum care should be arranged before delivery. Support is needed
to prevent relapse and to enhance mothering skills. The additional
physical and emotional strains of motherhood may frustrate the
heavy drinker and cause slips. Successful parenting requires complex skills, many of which are derived from attitudes and behaviors
learned early in life. Many alcoholics were raised in homes where
one or both parents abused alcohol. Deprived of good parenting,
they need help to master these skills.

Summary

Therapeutic intervention in all phases of problem drinking is effective when there is an alliance between the woman and the thera-
pist, focused on having a healthy child. It is extremely important
for pregnant women to establish and sustain relationships with
health professionals in which medical concern rather than a moralistic attitude predominates. Pregnancy is a normal crisis in a woman's life when changes in physiology, body image, and social role
cause her to think differently about herself. The sense of responsibility for another life increases many women's receptivity to help in
overcoming problem drinking.

Public health campaigns are useful in increasing the awareness
of the public about the risks of alcohol during pregnancy. However,
few alcoholics change their drinking patterns in response to mass
media campaigns (Pittman, 1980; Minor and Van Dort, 1982).
Obstetricians, family practitioners, pediatricians, and other health
professionals have the opportunity to intervene with positive results.
Women who drink heavily, whose children are at greatest risk, respond to individual supportive counselling provided by health care
professionals.

Nine

A Clinical Perspective

In the United States, approximately 5–10% of pregnant women drink at levels which may place the fetus at risk. On the basis of a population growth of 3.6 million births per year, 180,000 to 360,000 pregnancies are at risk for adverse outcome. These women represent all segments of society, the wealthy and the poor, the educated and the uneducated, and all ethnic groups. Effective prevention and treatment demand an understanding of alcohol and pregnancy by the entire health care delivery system. Women at risk and their families often require help with a range of problems in addition to counselling for heavy drinking during pregnancy.

Alcohol use before pregnancy

The ideal time to consider prevention of adverse effects of alcohol on the fetus is before the pregnancy begins. Prolonged heavy drinking interferes with the physiologic systems which are necessary for fertilization and conception as well as for optimal growth and development of the fetus (see Chapter 2). Information on the effects of heavy alcohol consumption on the endocrine system and reproductive functions of both male and female should be included when treating patients who are considering having a child.

EFFECTS ON THE MALE

Chronic alcohol consumption disrupts spermatogenesis by multiple direct and indirect mechanisms. Alcohol's interference with the production of testosterone reduces sperm levels. In addition, alcohol-related deficiencies in zinc and vitamin A associated with alcohol abuse and elevated blood acetaldehyde levels are deleterious to spermatogenesis. Reduced spermatogenesis decreases the likelihood of fertilization. However, when conception does occur, it is not clear what further effects of paternal alcohol abuse there are.

Clinical reports of paternal drinking and pregnancy outcome are fragmentary and inconclusive. In a survey of over 300 FAS cases, Abel (1982a) found mention of the father in only 38. Few epidemiologic studies have examined the effects of paternal alcohol consumption. Lemoine et al's (1968) reports of 127 children of alcoholic parents included 15 born to couples in which only the father was alcoholic, 25 with alcoholic mothers, and 29 with both parents alcoholic. Dysmorphology was greatest when the mother was alcoholic. A later, better-controlled prospective study by Kuzma and Sokol (1982) found no significant effects of paternal alcohol intake on infant birthweight.

Experimental research has been conducted on the potential for paternal drinking to damage sperm and to affect pregnancy outcome. Direct effects of chronic alcohol consumption on testicular spermatogoneal cells have been studied in the rat (Kohila et al, 1976). Rats who received a nutritionally adequate diet containing 10% ethanol for 70 days demonstrated no differences in the frequency of aberrations such as chromosomal breaks, chromatid breaks, and chromatid gaps. Subsequently, the experiment was repeated with male rats who received a thiamine-deficient diet as well as ethanol (Halkka and Eriksson, 1977). Again, there was no significant increase in chromosomal aberrations.

Badr and Badr (1975) found dominant lethal mutations at several spermatogenic stages following alcohol exposure. Ethanol was administered in doses of 1.24 and 1.88 g/kg by gastric tube to male mice for three consecutive days. Females mated 4–13 days after alcohol treatment of the male had a two- to four-fold increase in the number of dead implants.

Klassen and Persaud (1976) observed increased resorptions among offspring of alcohol-fed males. Six male rats fed an ethanol diet for five weeks became lethargic and ataxic, lost weight, and had ruffled, dull hair and small pale eyes. After five weeks, they had significantly lower blood sugar and testosterone levels than did the controls. After 15 days on the diet, each male was mated with two normally fed females on a nightly basis. When alcohol was withheld during hours of mating, withdrawal symptoms were observed. Among 13 females mated with controls, there were 158 pups and 9 early resorptions, while among 6 mated with the alcohol-fed males, there were 21 pups and 28 early resorptions. No malformed pups were observed, but pups of alcohol-fed fathers demonstrated significantly lower ($p < 0.01$) weight, length, and placental index, and lower growth index ($p < 0.5$).

Anderson et al (1978) observed reductions in average litter size among female mice mated with ethanol treated males. Tanaka et al (1982a) found decreased litter size as well as abnormalities in the progeny of alcohol-treated male rats. In contrast, Randall et al (1982) did not find any effects of paternal alcohol treatment on fetal growth and development in the mouse, including the number of implantation sites, prenatal mortality, fetal weight, sex ratio, or soft tissue malformations. Bennett et al (1982) reported similar outcomes. The discrepancies may reflect inadequate nutritional controls in the earlier studies, differences in the route of alcohol administration and blood alcohol levels, or species sensitivity.

In summary, clinical data on the effects of paternal alcohol consumption is sparse. Experimental data does not consistently demonstrate that FAS or other effects are caused by paternal consumption of alcohol. A review of findings to date suggests that the adverse effects of male alcohol abuse would be the failure of spermatogenesis or failure of fertilization (Van Thiel and Gavaler, 1982). Genetic injury would cause lethal mutations and spontaneous abortions should fertilization occur.

In animals, decreased litter size results from an increase in resorption of defective fetuses rather than the spermatazoa's inability to fertilize. In humans, the analogous phenomenon would be an increased tendency for spontaneous abortion. Patterns of assortative mating in humans result in the likelihood that women who drink heavily are impregnated by men who drink heavily. Paternal alcohol consumption has not been investigated in epidemiologic studies of the incidence of spontaneous abortion but it may have a causal role.

EFFECTS ON THE FEMALE

Maternal alcohol consumption may interfere with fertility and conception. Sandor et al (1980) reported decreased litter size in rats and mice exposed to 30% alcohol derived calories during preimplantation. Postimplantation exposure to the same doses was more harmful. Reports of alcoholic women who have stopped drinking prior to conception and have had normal children suggest that there are no relationships between pre-pregnancy drinking and neonatal outcome (Sullivan, 1899; Dehaene et al, 1977b; Olegård et al, 1977; Seidenberg and Majewski, 1978; Korányi and Csiky, 1978; Poskitt et al, 1982). One survey of pregnant women noted a relationship between infant status and maternal alcohol use pre-pregnancy, but not use during early pregnancy (Hanson et al, 1978). The authors suggest that it is difficult for women to differentiate alcohol consumption before conception from that before recognition of pregnancy. The association of alcohol use and adverse outcome probably results from consumption during the first stages of pregnancy. The single case of an FAS child born to a woman who had stopped drinking one and a half years prior to conception has been contested as not meeting the minimal criteria of FAS (Scheiner et al, 1979; Véghelyi, 1979; Smith and Graham, 1979).

Although adverse effects of alcohol abuse prior to conception have not been observed, pre-pregnancy sobriety is advisable to provide a period of physiologic, sociologic, and psychologic restitution. Recovery requires more than mere withdrawal; time is needed to change one's lifestyle. Social heavy drinkers often are able to abstain with support and encouragement from husband, family, and friends. Women drinking for symptom relief need to find new methods for dealing with anxiety and depression and may require counselling or psychotherapy. Alcohol-dependent women have a physiologic tolerance for alcohol and frequently have developed medical complications secondary to alcohol use. In addition, their lifestyle and social relationships have focused around alcohol use. Many require sustained support and specialized therapy. (See Chapter 8 for a discussion of treatment strategies.)

The recommended duration of sobriety prior to conception depends on the severity of the alcohol abuse. Women who have had medical complications of alcoholism such as hepatitis, pancreatitis, neuritis, or alterations in endocrine functioning should abstain for a year for optimal recovery. Women who have been drinking less heavily or for a brief period would require less time to stabilize. Both the father and the mother also should have time to adapt to the idea of parenthood and the acceptance of new responsibilities. Many couples may not delay conception because of other priorities in their lives. However, they should recognize that both potency and fertility will improve with sobriety.

Birth control for the alcoholic woman requires consideration of her ability to comply as well as her physiologic state. Alcohol has not been shown to have direct effects on the action of birth control pills, the diaphragm, or IUD. However, chronic alcoholism can alter the menstrual cycle and reduces the effectiveness of techniques which are based on the date of ovulation. Impulsivity and confusion caused by drinking can interfere with reliable use of methods such as the diaphragm or birth control pill.

There is no evidence that women who are drinking lightly need to abstain prior to conception. Needless stress can be created by excessive preoccupation with the dangers of small amounts of alcohol. The effort to conceive can be stressful in and of itself and should not be intensified by unnecessary changes in lifestyle. A female physician (Leak, 1983) who abstained from alcohol during the second half of each menstrual cycle found herself depressed after 12 months of trying to conceive. She felt that abstention increased the stress. She became pregnant four months after she resumed her normal lifestyle, including her consumption of approximately 10 drinks a week. During pregnancy, she experienced no further desire for alcohol. She believed that tension had interfered with her ability to conceive.

Alcohol use during pregnancy

PATTERNS OF CONSUMPTION

Some women should not drink any alcohol during pregnancy. Foremost are those with a vulnerability to addictive behavior. All women who report consuming 5 or more drinks on an occasion should be advised to stop drinking. Supportive counselling should be focused on abstaining for the remainder of the pregnancy. Women with a past history of addiction to alcohol or other substances should also be considered at risk. Advice to abstain from all drugs during pregnancy should be supplemented with help for any psychological and social problems which might increase stress and intensify the desire to drink.

The literature on the treatment of alcoholism contains an extensive debate on the possibility or advisability of controlled drinking. Total abstinence should be the goal for the pregnant recovering alcoholic to minimize the danger of relapse with its potential risk to the fetus. The time-limited duration of the pregnancy combined with the motivation to have a healthy child helps the alcoholic sustain abstinence.

For women with a vulnerability to addiction, caution is required when prescribing any medications. Sedatives should not be used as a substitute for alcohol consumption. Drugs to reduce anxiety or insomnia or to relieve withdrawal symptoms should be prescribed in the smallest effective dose for a strictly limited time.

Women with a physiologic vulnerability to adverse effects from alcohol should also abstain. A variety of medical complications contraindicate alcohol consumption during pregnancy. Clearly, women with a recent history of hepatitis or pancreatitis should not consume alcohol. Diabetic patients are more prone to ketoacidosis in the presence of alcohol. Women whose skin flushes after small amounts of alcohol may develop high acetaldehyde concentrations which are potentially teratogenic. Women requiring medications should be aware that the teratogenic properties of drugs may be potentiated by alcohol. (These issues are considered in more detail below.)

Responses to systematic questions about alcohol use may suggest the clinical recommendation of abstinence. Women who answer evasively or ambiguously may be defending against acknowledging problems controlling alcohol use. Women who ask excessively about the adverse effects of alcohol and are preoccupied with possible health consequences may have an obsessional desire to attain absolute health and safety. A woman who persists in asking for the most conservative and safest possible approach should be told that there is no danger from not drinking at all.

Women who consume 3 or 4 drinks on an occasion should be advised that this may represent a small risk which has not been determined at this time. Due to the uncertainties, drinking in this range should be discontinued for the duration of the pregnancy.

When there is no history of addictive behavior with alcohol or other drugs and no medical contraindications to alcohol use, danger from light drinking (less than 1 oz AA a day) has not been demonstrated and should not be overstated. Exaggeration will decrease the credibility concerning the established adverse effects of heavy drinking. Exaggerating the dangers may also create unnecessary guilt in the event of fetal abnormalities which could be caused by many other possible factors.

MEDICAL COMPLICATIONS

Problem drinkers are not less likely than others to receive prenatal care (Sokol et al, 1980; Weiner et al, 1983; Larsson, 1983). At Boston City Hospital, there were no differences among drinking groups in registration for prenatal care before the third trimester, although more heavy drinkers registered for prenatal care in the second than in the first trimester. Thirty-one women delivered with no prenatal care or registered after the 38th week: 8 were heavy drinkers, 7 were moderate, and 16 rare. This represented 5%, 1%, and 2% of the respective drinking groups.

Sokol et al (1980) observed an increased incidence of obstetrical complications in 204 women clinically identified as abusing alcohol. Among a cohort of 12,127 pregnancies, the alcohol abusing group was twice as likely to have received prenatal care in a special high-risk unit and to have required a nondelivery hospital admission. First and second trimester vaginal bleeding occurred almost three times more often. The risks of infection during delivery and of premature placental separation were increased. Fetal distress during labor and neonatal depression were more common. Seidenberg and Majewski (1978) observed bleeding and threatened abortion in 40% of alcoholic pregnant women compared with 12% of the population as a whole. Streissguth et al (1982) reported increases during labor and delivery in temperature, amnionitis, preeclampsia, and bleeding among women drinking at a "risk-level."

Chronic heavy alcohol consumption adversely affects almost every organ system in the body. Diseases of the liver and other parts of the gastrointestinal system, the cardiovascular system, and the hematopoietic system, as well as impairment of the body's defense mechanisms against infectious disease can complicate pregnancy. Alcohol can induce metabolic disturbances in the mother such as hypoglycemia, ketoacidosis, and alterations in lactate, uric acid, lipids, or individual amino acids.

Alcohol ketoacidosis is an infrequent but serious complication of pregnancy which can develop when heavy drinkers discontinue or reduce ethanol and food intake. The syndrome includes severe keto-acidosis, hyperpnea, normal glucose levels, absent glucosuria, and dehydration (Jenkins et al, 1971). Ovarian and placental hormones as well as the fetal drain on maternal carbohydrate reserves con-tribute to its pathogenesis. Careful medical management of keto-acidosis improves the prognosis for fetal survival. Treatment is di-rected toward fluid balance, correcting the electrolyte disturbance, and modifying abnormal carbohydrate metabolism.

Cooperman et al (1974) described severe ketoacidosis in six nondiabetic patients, one of whom was pregnant. She was admitted as an in-patient because of metabolic acidosis four times during two pregnancies. Each episode followed excessive drinking and each time the metabolic acidosis was progressively more severe. During the initial episode, she delivered a premature fetus at 30 weeks ges-tation. In her second pregnancy, she was admitted at 8, 28, and 32 weeks. This pregnancy produced a normal term infant.

Podratz (1978) also described a case of alcoholic ketoacidosis in pregnancy. The 23-year-old woman presented to the emergency room complaining of nausea and vomiting. She was dehydrated and suffering from acute respiratory distress. Initial management con-sisted of rapid fluid replacement, reversal of fatty acid mobilization, oxidation, neutralization of hydrogen ions and electrolyte balance. The patient responded favorably. Subsequently, a male SGA infant was delivered by caesarean section. Postoperative progress of both mother and baby was unremarkable, suggesting fetal ability to tol-erate low maternal arterial ph values and elevated serum ketone levels. Mental and motor development could not be followed as the child unfortunately suffered sudden infant death in his fifth week of life.

Two cases of severe ketoacidosis were identified in pregnant women at Boston City Hospital. The first woman was hospitalized on the medical service for severe gastroenteritis. She had not been a problem drinker, but with the onset of amenorrhea she had begun consuming a pint of liquor and six cans of beer a day. Since she had not been able to conceive during five years of marriage, she interpreted the cessation of menstruation as a sign of uterine cancer, which she dreaded. Acidosis and electrolyte disturbance were diagnosed, and an unsuspected pregnancy, 22 weeks by dates, was revealed. The fetus was 18 weeks by size with no heart beat. Autopsy was not performed following delivery at 29 weeks.

The second patient reported drinking one pint of liquor daily with binges on some weekends when she registered for prenatal care at 14 weeks. Her appetite was poor and weight gain during pregnancy was limited. At week 22, ketones were found in her urine and she was hospitalized. She quickly stabilized. Following abstention from alcohol, her appetite improved and there was a consistent weight gain. She delivered a normal sized baby at 39 weeks, weighing 2940 grams. Apgar scores were 2 and 8 at 1 and 5 minutes. Newborn examination was normal.

Chronic alcoholic women with advanced disease including Laennec cirrhosis rarely become pregnant. Crépin et al (1977) reviewed 20,000 deliveries over an 8-year period and found only 3 cases of alcoholic cirrhosis. All were associated with major complications of the pregnancy, and the offspring showed severe growth retardation and morphologic abnormalities. Alcoholic cirrhosis is the most frequent type, yet in another survey of 117 pregnancies in 92 patients with various types of cirrhosis, only 5 cases were identified (Cheng, 1977). This suggests that when the pathophysiologic changes of chronic alcoholism reach this stage, the woman's fertility and reproductive functions are so severely compromised that pregnancy rarely occurs.

RISK FACTORS

Heavy drinking often is associated with other variables that contribute to reproductive risk, such as nutritional deficiency, heavy smoking, use of other drugs, and emotional stress. The interaction between these associated factors and alcohol is briefly considered below. While each of these factors places the woman at risk, sustained heavy drinking represents an independent and important hazard to fetal growth and development.

Nutrition. Poor dietary intake, disturbances of intermediate metabolism, impaired intestinal absorption, elevated urinary loss, gastrointestinal disturbances, and hepatic damage affect the nutritional status of the chronic alcoholic. At Boston City Hospital, the heavy-drinking women did not report significantly different dietary intake than the rare and moderate drinkers (Rosett et al, 1978). However, few patients met the minimum daily requirements of the National Research Council. Impaired utilization among the heavy drinkers further limits nutritional status. Specific impairment of the active transport of essential amino acids across the placenta causes selective malnutrition of the fetus. In addition, heavy alcohol use impairs synthesis of essential fatty acids (Horrobin, 1980).

The association of multiple nutritional deficiencies with fetal maldevelopment underscores the need for sobriety throughout pregnancy. Supplementary minerals and vitamins may help restore the depleted supplies. However, these are of little value as long as abusive drinking continues, and they should not be considered an alternative to abstinence.

Recent animal research on supplements may hold promise for future treatment strategies. Varma and Persaud (1982) experimentally administered primrose oil and high doses of alcohol to pregnant rats. Primrose oil is rich in several essential fatty acids, including linoleic and gamma-linolenic, which are necessary for the synthesis of various neurochemicals. Growth retardation did not occur in rats fed primrose oil and alcohol, but did occur in those exposed to equivalent doses of alcohol alone. Tanaka et al (1982c) also demonstrated that fetal development was less disturbed when zinc or glucose was administered with the experimental ethanol, although it did not reach the level of the controls.

Cigarettes. The association between heavy drinking and heavy cigarette smoking has been consistently observed in seven epidemiologic studies of pregnancy in the United States, Canada, and France (Weiner et al, 1983). In the survey at our prenatal clinic, 53% of the heavy drinkers smoked over 10 cigarettes per day while only 14% of the rare drinkers smoked in this range. Stepwise multiple regression analysis demonstrated that cigarette smoking and heavy drinking each accounted for a statistically significant amount of the variance in birthweight and length (Rosett et al, 1983b). When analysis focused on babies who were small for gestational age, heavy drinking was the strongest predictor. Cigarette and/or marijuana smoking without sustained heavy drinking did not increase the risk of having an SGA baby. In contrast, Sokol et al (1980) found that the risk of SGA was increased 2.4-fold in association with alcohol abuse alone, 1.8-fold with smoking alone, and 3.9-fold with the combined risks. Longo (1977) reviewed the effects of cigarette smoking and found increased perinatal mortality, congenital heart disease, and complications of pregnancy such as abruptio placenta, placenta previa, and premature rupture of fetal membranes. The multiple components of cigarette smoke were investigated, particularly carbon monoxide. However, the data was not adjusted for alcohol consumption.

Reductions in cigarette smoking during pregnancy have been observed, but have not been so marked as reductions in alcohol use. Fried et al (1980) reported an 8% reduction in cigarettes and 66% reduction in the use of alcohol. Kuzma and Kissinger (1980) observed that 4.7% stopped smoking cigarettes for 1 or 2 trimesters while 11.4% abstained from alcohol. Clinical programs to help women reduce cigarette use during pregnancy have not been encouraging (Landesman-Dwyer and Emanuel, 1979).

Experimental studies have not demonstrated an interaction between alcohol and nicotine on fetal growth and development. Prenatal exposure of rats to 6 g/kg per day of alcohol plus nicotine did not have a more adverse effect than exposure to alcohol alone (Abel et al, 1979). Acute and chronic exposure of rats to moderate doses of ethanol plus nicotine had no significant adverse effects on embryonic development (Persaud, 1982; Lindenschmidt and Persaud, 1980).

Caffeine. Coffee consumption is associated with use of both alcohol and cigarettes. Among 12,000 pregnant women, caffeine consumption increased in direct relationship to alcohol intake and cigarette smoking (Kuzma and Kissinger, 1981). While there is an association between alcohol and coffee consumption, there is no evidence that coffee consumption causes growth retardation or malformations. Animal studies that have implicated caffeine as a teratogen have employed very large doses—the equivalent of 40 to 100 cups of coffee per day (Mulvihill, 1973). In addition, the fetus may be protected by a rapid metabolism of caffeine, with only 1% secreted unchanged (Gilbert, 1976).

No associations were found between coffee consumption and pregnancy outcomes among 12,400 women when the data was controlled for smoking and previous pregnancy history (Linn et al,

1982). Similarly, no effects of coffee drinking were observed among 1690 infant–mother pairs examined postpartum at Boston City Hospital (Hingson et al, 1982). A study of 482 defective children and matched controls also found no relationships between maternal coffee consumption and children's status (Kurpa et al, 1982).

Drugs. Many different classes of drugs and medications can affect fetal development (Hill, 1978). Alcohol has at least an additive effect with most other drugs and potentiates many of them. An annotated bibliography of this subject lists 1500 references (Polacsek et al, 1972) and extensive reviews have been published (Kissin, 1974; Deitrich and Petersen, 1979). The pharmacokinetics of the interaction between alcohol and other drugs can increase risks to the fetus when women drink heavily while using other agents. In addition, the induction of microsomal drug metabolizing enzymes in chronic alcoholics may increase the teratogenic effects of licit and illicit drugs.

Adverse effects of psychoactive drug use by males and females on reproduction and fetal development have been reviewed by Joffe and Soyka (1982) and by Finnegan and Fehr (1980). Prospective studies demonstrate associations between heavy drinking and the use of psychoactive drugs during pregnancy. At Boston City Hospital, 3–4% of the women who reported heavy drinking in the prenatal survey acknowledged use of heroin, barbiturates, psychedelics, or amphetamines (Weiner et al, 1983). This was significantly greater than among the moderate and rare drinkers, less than 1% of whom acknowledged using these substances. The small number of identified users may account for the lack of a statistical relationship between the use of any drugs and fetal maldevelopment.

Marijuana was the most commonly used drug. In the prenatal clinic, 31% of the women who drank heavily reported at the time of registration that they had smoked marijuana compared with 18% of the moderate drinkers and 9% of the rare drinkers (Rosett et al, 1983b). When mothers were surveyed on the Boston City Hospital obstetrical service following delivery, 43% of the heavy drinkers reported that they had smoked marijuana during pregnancy, compared with 14% of the total population (Hingson et al, 1982). Among the women interviewed both prenatally and postpartum, 35 reported marijuana use during pregnancy at both interviews. An additional 35 reported use during pregnancy either at registration or postpartum. Discrepant reports of marijuana use may reflect denial or changes in smoking patterns. Exposure late in pregnancy may have a greater effect on the fetus. Marijuana smoking during pregnancy as reported postdelivery was statistically related to reduction of mean birthweight, while use reported at prenatal clinic registration was not. Fried (1980) reported dose-related nervous system abnormalities and diminished visual responses among neonates exposed to marijuana in utero. Birthweight and gestational age did not differ. At one year, all symptoms had attenuated (Fried, 1982).

Fetal hydantoin syndrome, a pattern of congenital malformations, growth deficiency, and retarded mental development, which resembles FAS, has been observed in neonates exposed in utero to antiepileptic drugs. Congenital anomalies have been observed in association with prenatal use of the following anticonvulsants, alone or in combination: barbiturates, hydantoins, oxazolidines, succinimides, benzodiazepines, acetylurea, or carbamazepine (Janz, 1975). Long-term treatment with phenytoin, primidone, or phenobarbitol can disturb the metabolism of calcium, corticosteroids, folic acid, and vitamin D, as well as alter connecting tissue repair processes and prothrombin time (Hill, 1976). Similarities between the chronic effects of anticonvulsants and alcohol on maternal physiology and metabolism—and presumably on the fetus—may explain similarities in the abnormalities found in exposed offspring.

The synergistic effect of alcohol and hydantoin is suggested by case reports of infants born with extensive abnormalities following maternal use of both substances (Ramilo and Harris, 1979; Seeler et al, 1979; Wilker and Nathenson, 1982). Alcoholic women are more likely to be suffering from seizure disorders than are other pregnant women and therefore are more likely to require anticonvulsant medication. The risks of anticonvulsant medication must be weighed against the benefits of controlling seizures. When anticonvulsants are prescribed during pregnancy, the patient should be warned of the additional risks of alcohol consumption.

The benzodiazepines are frequently prescribed to control acute withdrawal from alcohol and to treat subsequent insomnia and anxiety. Their teratogenic potential has been suggested and may be increased with alcohol consumption (Kellogg et al, 1980). Benzodiazepines cause greater depression of the central nervous system when used in conjunction with alcohol than either agent does alone (Sellers and Busto, 1982). Plasma levels of diazepam are significantly higher following administration with ethanol than with water. Thus, in addition to an interaction between ethanol and diazepam in the CNS, ethanol may enhance absorption or inhibit the metabolism of the diazepam.

Simultaneous intake of ethanol with the psychotherapeutic agent chlorpromazine caused a 60% decrease in its rate of removal from rat blood (Rawat, 1980). Prolonged maternal ethanol consumption during pregnancy and lactation leads to a decrease in chlorpromazine metabolism in the fetal, neonatal, and maternal livers.

Solvents have been associated with congenital CNS defects (Holmberg, 1979). Exposure in combination with alcohol may potentiate the teratogenicity. The capacity to metabolize alcohol may be impaired by the solvents, while the alcohol may increase the toxicity of toluene. A child with "nearly classic" FAS was reported born to a mother who acknowledged toluene abuse and consumption of a six pack of beer weekly (Toutant and Lippman, 1979).

Medications may themselves become substances of abuse. A case was reported of a 24-year-old woman who gave birth to a child with signs of fetal alcohol effects after consuming 4–7 bottles of cough syrup daily during pregnancy (Chasnoff et al, 1981). The cough syrup contained 9.5% alcohol; her actual daily alcohol intake was equivalent to 3–5 drinks daily.

Stress. Heavy-drinking women are frequently using alcohol to relieve symptoms of depression and anxiety. The effects of maternal anxiety have been reported to be deleterious to rat offspring (Kellogg et al, 1980). Stress-induced chemical and endocrine alterations can disrupt the maternal-placental-fetal system. An increased level of epinephrine in the mother diverts blood from the uterus to other maternal organs, thereby decreasing the supply of oxygen to the fetus. Maternal fears and anxieties about pregnancy and other life events have been associated with infant morbidity. Complications observed in the neonate and child include pyloric stenosis (Revill and Dodge, 1978), behavior problems (Ferreira, 1960; Stott and Latchford, 1976), and irritability (Ottinger and Simmons, 1964). Differences have not been found among children of women with various psychiatric diagnoses; however, when psychiatric patients were divided on a dimension of chronicity, those with the greatest number of psychiatric contacts and hospitalizations had more infants with perinatal complications (Sameroff and Chandler, 1975).

Labor

INHIBITION OF PREMATURE LABOR

Intravenous ethanol has been used to arrest premature labor. The initial dose of 15 ml/kg per hour for two hours is followed by 1.5 ml/kg per hour for six additional hours or until labor subsides. BACs peak at approximately 178 mg percent (Caritis et al, 1979). At equivalent concentrations (100–160 mg percent), the release of oxytocin by the pituitary was inhibited (Fuchs et al, 1967) but there was no effect on the uterine muscle (Wagner and Fuchs, 1968; Wilson et al, 1969).

Since the dose of alcohol required to arrest labor often causes intoxication in the woman, nausea and vomiting are common side effects. More severe reactions have also been reported. Intravenous administration of alcohol during labor stimulated the acidity and volume of maternal gastric secretion. Subsequent administration of anesthesia was associated with aspirations of a highly acid secretion followed by pneumonitis (Greenhouse et al, 1969).

Risks to the fetus from intravenous alcohol have been identified experimentally and clinically. Maternal and fetal acid-base balance was disturbed in pregnant ewes treated with 15 ml/kg of body weight of 9.75% solution of ethanol for 1 or 2 hours (Mann et al, 1975a). The peak concentration in the maternal blood was 237 mg at 90 minutes and in the fetal blood was 222 mg percent at 120 minutes. Maternal hyperlactacidemia and hyperglycemia were noted, but there was no significant alteration of the maternal acid-base balance. Fetal metabolic acidosis and a mixed acidosis observed during the alcohol infusion worsened during the postinfusion period. Fetal EEG showed a decrease in amplitude and a slowing of the dominant rhythm as the BAC increased (Mann et al, 1975b). The EEG became isoelectric on occasion during the postinfusion period in association with severe fetal acidosis. Fetal cerebral oxygen uptake was unaffected, while the cerebral uptake of glucose and the glucose-oxygen utilization ratio was significantly increased. Horiguchi et al (1975) carried out similar investigations with 13 pregnant rhesus monkeys, with fetal ages ranging from 120 to 160 days (term is about 168 days). They were infused during 60 minutes with 2–4 g/kg ethanol after the spontaneous onset of labor or following its induction by oxytocin infusion. Maximum BACs were

237 mg percent. The maternal respiratory rate was decreased, and fetal heart rate increased. The authors also observed a fetal acidosis and concluded that intravenous infusion of ethanol in doses sufficient to suppress labor may be hazardous because the fetus becomes progressively asphyxiated.

Decreased cardiac contractility was observed in fetal sheep following maternal intubation with 15 cc/kg alcohol (Kirkpatrick et al, 1976). Maternal BACs reached an excess of 110 mg percent. Exposure to alcohol and hysterotomy occurred on gestational days 110–124. Cardiac evaluations were performed 14–30 days later, suggesting that alcohol intubation to postpone labor might depress myocardial performance in the neonate.

Clinical studies of ethanol treatment to arrest labor also suggest adverse fetal effects. Zervoudakis et al (1980) observed significantly greater risk among newborns whose mothers were treated with alcohol than among matched controls. Infants were matched for birthweight, gestational age, delivery date, intact maternal membranes at onset of labor, anesthesia, and delivery. Alcohol-exposed infants had an increased frequency of respiratory distress. Among alcohol-exposed infants who weighed 1001–1500 grams, there was increased infant mortality.

When premature labor ceases following intravenous alcohol administration, women have been advised to continue therapy with beverage alcohol. Doses which may be effective are in the range of six drinks per day. The resulting BAC could have direct adverse effects on the fetal CNS. The clinician must weigh these potential pathologic effects before prescribing ethanol to inhibit labor. Alternative treatments, including bed rest, have been found to be as effective as ethanol and should be considered (Abel, 1981b). Ritodrine hydrochloride was approved by the FDA in 1980 for use in halting premature labor (Barden et al, 1980; Merkatz et al, 1980).

OBSTETRICAL ANESTHESIA

Anesthetic management of the alcoholic patient is complex because of interactions between the effects of alcohol and those of the general anesthetic and premedication. In the acutely intoxicated patient, the excitatory induction phase of anesthesia is more prolonged and more violent. More anesthetic agent is needed to overcome the excitatory stage, but less is needed to produce deep narcosis because of the synergism between ethanol and anesthetics (Kissin, 1974). Abstinent chronic alcoholics have a greater tolerance for general anesthetic agents and require larger doses (Shibutani, 1971). In the pregnant alcoholic, interactions between alcohol and general anesthetics increase fetal risk. Administration of anesthesia to a woman who had been treated with intravenous alcohol caused aspirations of a highly acid secretion followed by pneumonitis (Greenhouse et al, 1969). In view of the unpredictable response of the mother and the fetus to general anesthesia, local anesthesia or natural childbirth procedures are indicated both for the chronic alcoholic and for women who have been drinking heavily prior to delivery.

Infancy

NEONATAL PERIOD

Acute withdrawal signs are rare following in utero exposure to alcohol. They have been observed only in neonates born to chronic alcoholic women who continued to drink heavily to term (Schaefer, 1962; Nichols, 1967). Pierog et al (1977) reported withdrawal signs in six infants who were subsequently diagnosed as FAS. The most prominent symptoms were irritability and tremor, startle reaction to noise, abdominal distention, and spontaneous convulsion. At Boston City Hospital, we did not observe neonatal withdrawal from alcohol. Neonates of women who abuse alcohol and other drugs are at risk for withdrawal seizures associated with opiate or sedative abstinence syndrome (Finnegan, 1979; Finnegan and Fehr, 1980). Close observation of these patients is warranted.

When a woman undergoes withdrawal in mid-pregnancy, it seems probable that the fetus would be subject to major metabolic and physiologic disturbances. Two patients who had been consuming over a quart of vodka a day were withdrawn during the second trimester on the Boston City Hospital Obstetrical Service (Rosett and Weiner, 1981). They were given decreasing amounts of alcohol for one week to modify withdrawal symptoms. No adverse effects were detected in monitoring fetal heart rate or on careful neurologic examination of the newborn.

SLEEP STATE

Newborns of problem drinkers have demonstrated alterations in sleep patterns (see Chapter 4). Disturbances in an infant's regulation of sleep state may have far-reaching detrimental effects on the quality of mother–child interaction. The basic temporal organization of the neonate's nervous system develops through interacting with the caregiver during the first weeks of life. A baby who sleeps regularly and eats and naps at predictable times is far easier to care for than one with an erratic schedule, who remains a frustrating mystery to the mother. If the mother is also drinking heavily and has limited tolerance for frustration, the possibility of disturbed interaction between mother and child is great. Her frustrations during the baby's first weeks of life may intensify the mother's sense of failure as a caregiver and initiate a vicious cycle in which her self-esteem lessens and early bonding suffers. Thus, what is initially a physiologic disturbance may result in a sustained behavioral problem. The mother should understand the physiologic component and be taught techniques for comforting the restless and irritable baby, which might help regulate and calm it. Infants with sleep disturbances often respond favorably to dark and quiet sleeping areas, attention to the timing of interventions, swaddling, eye contact, and a soothing voice, all of which contribute to a more satisfying attachment between the mother and infant.

BREAST FEEDING

Alcohol reaches the same concentration in the nursing mother's breast milk as in her blood. However, since the volume of milk consumed during a feeding interval is further diluted throughout the infant's total body water, the infant's BAC will be much lower. There are approximately 2.4 liters of body water in a 4 kg (8.8 lb) infant. An average feeding contains about 100 ml of milk. If this is provided by an intoxicated mother with a BAC of 150 mg percent, the infant will ingest 150 mg of alcohol. This is diluted throughout 2.4 liters, resulting in an infant BAC of 6.3 mg percent. Oxidization occurs at a much slower rate in the infant than in the adult since the hepatic alcohol dehydrogenase is not fully active.

Physiologic effects and the rate of excretion have not been studied systematically in the infant. However, the low BAC resulting from a single drink would seem to be of little concern. The effects of a single episode of intoxication probably are limited to mild sedation. Chronic exposure to high doses of alcohol is potentially dangerous. Actively alcoholic women should not breast feed. Advice to drink beer to promote milk production should be given cautiously since it can be interpreted by some women as permission to consume large quantities. A single case report of "pseudo-Cushing" syndrome has been reported in a baby breast-fed by a mother who drank "at least 50 12-ounce cans of beer weekly, plus generous amounts of other more concentrated alcoholic drinks" (Binkiewicz et al, 1978). When the mother stopped drinking, the baby's symptoms disappeared.

Childhood and adolescence

POSTNATAL GROWTH RETARDATION

Postnatal growth retardation is of great concern to parents, and often is the primary complaint when FAS children are presented for diagnostic evaluation. In most instances, growth retardation has a pathophysiologic basis and will persist despite adequate nutrition and an appropriate environment. Multiple endocrine and nutritional investigations may be normal and not explain the growth failure. FAS children present specific feeding problems because of their poor sucking ability and malformations of the oral pharynx. Allowing the child more time to eat and being careful about the size of the portions may make eating easier for these children, but will not always improve growth. Alcohol's role in growth retardation should be explained to parents to facilitate their acceptance of the fact that their small child will probably be a small adult.

DEVELOPMENTAL DELAYS

Reports on the most severely damaged children have resulted in a pessimistic prognosis for the intellectual development of all children with FAS. Biological hazards are most likely to lead to later sequelae when they are combined with psychosocial adversity. Long-term studies of children impaired by other perinatal factors such as anoxia and prematurity suggest that a stimulating environment improves developmental outcome (Drillien, 1964; Sameroff and Chandler, 1975). Children with milder forms of FAS respond to early stimulation and tutoring in a facilitating environment (Bierich, 1978; Koranyi and Csiky, 1978; Steinhausen et al, 1982). Any special interests or talents that are demonstrated should be fostered. Reviewing the child's potential areas of learning and social adaptation helps parents adopt realistic expectations. Periodic conferences can call attention to the child's progress and mastery both in academic areas and in tasks of living.

In the absence of FAS, the clinical link between in utero exposure to alcohol and developmental problems is difficult to establish. A systematic history of maternal drinking should be part of an extensive attempt to identify etiology. There is no evidence that consumption of less than 1 oz AA per day damages the fetus. Parents of abnormal children who experience guilt because they were drinking these amounts should be reassured. When heavy drinking is identified, it should be treated as an obstacle to effective parenting even if its role as the cause of damage may not be established.

BEHAVIORAL PROBLEMS

Children of alcoholics are a high-risk group for many behavioral problems, including hyperactivity, delinquency, and alcoholism (Cork, 1969; Chafetz et al, 1971; Goodwin et al, 1973; El-Guebaly and Offord, 1977). This pessimistic prognosis is undoubtedly multidetermined. Genetic components to affective disorders have been described (Goodwin, 1971). The environment in a family where one or both parents is alcoholic may not provide the stability and consistency necessary for successful child rearing (Jackson, 1954). Alcohol-induced changes in the developing CNS may contribute to both behavioral aberrations and alcoholism.

Rats exposed to alcohol in utero were hyperactive and consumed significantly more ethanol in preference tests than did controls (Bond and DiGiusto, 1976). This finding led the authors to question whether hyperactivity and alcoholism are associated. Alcohol-induced changes in the hypothalamic-pituitary axis which affect the rat's response to stress also might predispose to alcoholism (Taylor et al, 1983). While experimental research suggests that children exposed to alcohol in utero might suffer an excessive incidence of alcoholism, longitudinal studies are needed to clarify this issue.

The family

Therapy of heavy drinking which begins during pregnancy should continue postpartum. Abstinence or moderation of alcohol consumption can be bolstered by a supportive and educational approach concerning parenthood which continues through the first years of the baby's life. Since regular contact with the obstetrician usually diminishes after delivery, involvement of other health professionals should be initiated during the third trimester. Referrals must be coordinated to assure continuity of care for the mother and child.

Support is particularly important when the child demonstrates adverse effects from alcohol exposure. Professionals have been reluctant to discuss the diagnosis of FAS even when the signs are apparent. They dread confronting the parents with the evidence that maternal alcohol abuse caused the child's disabilities, fearing that this will create guilt and lead to increased alcoholism and neglect of the child. Even when the mother has been drinking in secret, she knows that she has been drinking heavily. She feels that she has fallen short of her expectations for ideal mothering. She experiences guilt but has no one with whom she can share it. Her attempts to undo guilt may lead to repetitive medical work-ups of the child in which the essential information about alcohol consumption is omitted. In her frustration, she may drink more and become depressed. Direct discussion of the facts in a nonmoralistic fashion can bring relief and free her to devote her energy toward alcoholism treatment for herself and remedial programs for the child. Finkelstein et al (1981) reduced maternal guilt by helping women recognize that they and their families were victims of alcoholism and that inappropriate behavior while drinking was neither deliberately malicious nor voluntary. Peer support groups helped alcoholic mothers accept the idea that options were limited during periods of active drinking, and enabled them to forgive themselves and gradually accept the responsibilities of motherhood.

Once the diagnosis of FAS has been established, outreach should be made to all family members. Heavy alcohol consumption by the

mother often is associated with heavy drinking by the father. Treatment of the father's drinking problem will help him accept himself,
his wife, and his children. While evidence of adverse effects on
children from paternal drinking is inconclusive, there is strong evidence that alcohol abuse by either parent interferes with childrear-
ing and is detrimental to development.

The role of the father during infancy has been the subject of
considerable recent investigation (Parke, 1979). The father is an
important member of the family and plays an active and distinctive
role in the infant's social, emotional, and cognitive development.
Both the quantity and quality of the interactions between father
and infant have been shown to have significant effects. Paternal attitudes and actions also influence the mother's behavior with the
infant.

In a family where both parents drink heavily, there is a tendency
for each parent to blame the other, projecting their guilt and frustration. The therapeutic goal for each of the parents should be abstinence. As they both obtain mastery over their alcoholism they
will be able to accept themselves as well as their spouse and their
children and provide a more stable love object for the child. Alcoholic fathers often have difficulty controlling their rage and withdraw
from the parenting role in order to avoid physically abusing their
children (Mayer et al, 1978). They make a deliberate decision not to
discipline their children while they are drinking and fail to provide
consistent limits. The physiologic toll of alcohol abuse hinders the
successful completion of the emotional and physical tasks of motherhood (DeElejalde, 1971). The moods and physical state of the alcoholic mother vary greatly and so do her responses to her child. She
has difficulty with time-oriented tasks and often cannot cope with
children's daily needs.

Summary

Proper management of heavy-drinking women and their progeny
requires an understanding of the multiple compounding risk factors and the importance of a continuum of care. The prenatal period
may be complicated by illnesses and other reproductive hazards. In
the infant exposed to alcohol in utero, irritability, difficulty feeding,
and irregular sleep may contribute to the mother's neglect rather

than result from poor mothering. Psychological and social stresses of the familial environment exacerbate the problems that result from alcohol-induced damage to the CNS, further impeding the child's development. A pessimistic prognosis for FAS children has developed, based on reports on the most severe cases. However, children with milder fetal alcohol effects can respond to remedial efforts in a stable, supportive environment.

Ten

Strategies for Prevention

Determining health policy

Clinical and experimental findings on alcohol and pregnancy have been evaluated by individual researchers and by scientific councils and organizations. Data has been carefully scrutinized in an attempt to determine what we do and don't know about alcohol's effects during pregnancy. Many of the methodologic limitations have been considered. Although the discipline and focus have varied among reviewers, the scientific conclusions have been largely consistent. Interpretations of the data for health policy have differed.

Reviews of the experimental literature have demonstrated dose responses (Rosett, 1980b). Behavioral and morphological effects occur when alcohol concentrations are equivalent to the clinical level of intoxication. Randall (1982) concluded that anomalies were observed in association with BACs in excess of 100 mg percent. Abel and Greizerstein (1982) estimate that 150 mg percent is the minimal level associated with growth retardation. Bond (1981) stated in a review of behavioral teratogenesis that adverse effects were seen in association with doses of at least 6–7 g/kg per day.

Neugut (1981) appraised the epidemiologic literature and concluded that there was overwhelming evidence that in utero exposure to heavy doses of alcohol was associated with untoward pregnancy outcome. However, she felt that none of the studies adequately supported the proposition that in utero alcohol alone was the causative factor. More rigorous data analysis was required, especially in the area of intellectual development.

Reports on FAS and FAE have been included in Special Reports on Alcohol and Health from the Secretary of Health and Human Services to the U.S. Congress. The first discussion of alcohol and pregnancy appeared in 1978, in the Third Special Report. The evidence from a comprehensive review of early clinical and experimental studies was described as compelling (USDHEW, 1978). Risks to the fetus were observed when daily alcohol consumption exceeded 3 oz (6 drinks). As a result of the report, health-care providers were advised to warn against consumption of more than 1–2 drinks a day during pregnancy.

The Fourth Special Report on Alcohol and Health, presented to the U.S. Congress in 1981, also included a report on fetal alcohol effects (USDHHS, 1981). After reviewing recent research, the authors concluded: "A rapidly growing body of literature provides evidence that abusive drinking during pregnancy is potentially detrimental to development of the human fetus. Effects may range from mild physical and behavioral deficits to the FAS." Heavier alcohol use during pregnancy was also associated with decreased birthweight, spontaneous abortions, and adverse behavioral and neurological effects on newborns. The authors thought that several issues required further research, including the effects of low doses, individual susceptibility, and vulnerable gestational periods.

On the basis of this report, the Surgeon General issued an advisory (Surgeon General, 1981) stating, "A woman who consumes alcohol at amounts consistent with the diagnosis of alcoholism risks bearing a child with the specific cluster of severe physical and mental defects known as Fetal Alcohol Syndrome. Health professionals are urged to inquire routinely about alcohol consumption by patients who are pregnant or considering pregnancy." He further advised women who are pregnant (or considering pregnancy) not to drink alcoholic beverages and "to be aware of the alcoholic content of food and drugs." This last phrase implies that the smallest amount of alcohol may be detrimental to fetal development. With the exception of the three papers cited by the Surgeon General (Little, 1977; Kline et al, 1980; Harlap and Shiono, 1980), few studies support the recommendation of total abstinence. The evidence that small amounts of alcohol have adverse effects on pregnancy has been debated (Kolata, 1981; Rosett and Weiner, 1982). Attempts to replicate these studies have failed. What is appropriate advice to give to pregnant women remains controversial.

Fabro (1979) comprehensively reviewed both animal and clinical research programs as part of a public awareness campaign by the Department of the Treasury and the Bureau of Alcohol, Tobacco, and Firearms. In response to the question of whether or not a minimum "safe" level existed, he stated that a clear relationship between alcohol use and pregnancy outcome was demonstrated only for heavy and prolonged maternal alcohol abuse. The effects of lower levels are questionable. Although a numerical value for a safe pattern could not be specified, he concluded that it is likely that there is a level of alcohol consumption that is not associated with toxicity. Until more data is accumulated, he advised pregnant women to abstain from alcohol.

In a later review, Fabro (1982) concluded that there were few experimental studies which demonstrated effects below 2 g/kg per day. He further observed that, in humans, alcohol's adverse effects on fetal development follow a dose-response relationship standard for teratogens. Although no-effect levels have not been established and may differ depending on outcome variable studied, drinking patterns, and genetics, he saw no evidence of any adverse effects associated with light alcohol consumption (0.5 oz AA per day).

The American Council of Science and Health (ACSH) (1981) extensively reviewed the scientific evidence and concluded that the consumption of large amounts of alcohol is clearly hazardous to fetal development. The Council further stated that although no safe levels of alcohol ingestion have been defined or ever would be, the health risks associated with small amounts are low, if they exist at all. Women should be cautious about alcohol use during pregnancy. Those who choose to drink should limit alcohol intake to two drinks or less a day. While total abstinence is the safest course, ACSH was concerned that excessive health warnings might be counterproductive, equating hypothetical risks with real risks and thereby desensitizing women to all warnings.

The American Medical Association Council on Scientific Affairs (1983) also reviewed the body of scientific evidence and issued a report designed to increase physician awareness. The council agreed that pregnant women who drink heavily place their unborn child at risk. Physicians should be alert to signs of alcohol abuse among women of childbearing age and take appropriate diagnostic and therapeutic measures. There is a possibility of a dose-response phenomenon through which different levels of alcohol intake may be roughly associated with differing degrees and types of adverse outcomes. Fetal risks from moderate or minimal alcohol consumption are not established. Until more definitive information is available, physicians should inform patients what research does and does not show and encourage them to decide about drinking in light of the evidence and their own situations. Although there is not definitive research support of statements linking low doses with risk, the AMA suggests that physicians advise patients that abstinence is the safest course.

MEDIA CAMPAIGNS

Widespread recognition of alcohol's potential for adversely affecting both fetal development and the mother–infant relationship has stimulated the development of a variety of prevention programs. Campaigns have been sponsored by NIAAA and other federal agencies to increase the public's awareness of the effects of alcohol on pregnancy (U.S. Department of the Treasury, 1980; NIAAA Alcohol Abuse Prevention Campaign, 1982). Several state task forces have conducted education campaigns by distributing pamphlets in physicians' offices, liquor stores, and retail centers and presenting spot announcements on television and radio. Media campaigns have also been sponsored by private agencies, including the National Council on Alcoholism and the March of Dimes. These have been effective in increasing awareness in the general population (Opinion Research Corporation, 1979).

Women who drink heavily and whose children are at greatest risk are the least responsive to this type of campaign (Little et al, 1981). Not unexpectedly, a review of similar prevention programs indicated that public education does not reduce chronic alcoholism (Pittman, 1980). Despite women's awareness of the potential dangers of alcohol use during pregnancy, which a recent evaluation of women's attitudes and behavior revealed (Minor and Van Dort, 1982), 20% reported consumption at levels that they themselves defined as "risk." Fewer women who discussed alcohol use with their physicians continued risky drinking. When the smoking and drinking habits of women who were pregnant before public awareness of FAS were compared with those of pregnant women 6 years later, alcohol use was found to have decreased among rare and moderate

1 the number of abstainers had increased (Streissguth
There were no differences, however, in the percent of
on drinking heavily.

PROFESSIONAL EDUCATION

Seminars and symposia to educate health care professionals have
been sponsored by medical societies and public health agencies.
Material presented at some of these sessions has been disseminated
in professional journals. However, it has not been determined which
professionals attend the meetings or whether the information is incorporated into their clinical behavior.

At Boston City Hospital, we included information on alcohol and
pregnancy in the orientation program for interns and residents in
the obstetrical department (Weiner et al, 1982). The Ten Question
Drinking History (see Appendix), which was printed on the prenatal intake form, provided the house staff with a structured format
for inquiring about alcohol use. Use of the Ten Question Drinking
History, monitored for each of six study periods, varied. However,
throughout the study at least one third of the patients were asked
about alcohol use. This represents a marked increase in the number
of inquiries about drinking patterns. These training activities currently are being extended to include the range of health care professionals who provide services to women of childbearing age throughout Massachusetts.

In Seattle, a project was developed to raise the level of community awareness and to educate health care professionals (Little
et al, 1980). Formal presentations to physicians were supplemented
by publications in professional journals. Awareness among the obstetricians and frequency of advising patients on alcohol and pregnancy increased during the two-year period of the program (Little
et al, 1983). Most physicians recommended that alcohol use be limited to 1–2 drinks a day.

Realistic counselling

Professionals who counsel alcoholics primarily work with addicted
patients. Alcohol is the central issue, with total abstinence the ther-

apeutic goal. Clinicians who work with pregnant women must recognize multiple determinants of fetal outcome. Alcohol is one of many risk factors to be considered. They must encourage health habits in many areas of life which can be accepted and sustained throughout pregnancy. When the pregnant patient is an alcoholic or has had other problems with addictive behavior, total abstinence must be the goal. For all patients, clinical priorities must be based on an objective evaluation of a range of possible hazards to the fetus.

It is not possible to issue a simple recommendation appropriate for the entire population. In most medical decisions the clinician and the patient must assess the risks and benefits and decide on the best course of action. Because of the complexity and ambiguity associated with alcohol consumption and its effects on the fetus, the need for individual counselling is particularly great.

Advice should be consistent and sustained throughout the pregnancy and the neonatal period by all of the professionals who work with the woman and her child. Pregnant women have relationships with many health professionals—family practitioners, obstetricians, pediatricians caring for older children, nurses, midwives, social workers, nutritionists, and perhaps alcoholism counsellors. The messages she receives must be consistent if they are to have credibility. They should be based on facts, not exaggeration, to avoid one group of professionals disagreeing with and rejecting the advice of another group and thereby diminishing therapeutic effectiveness.

Review of the clinical and experimental evidence suggests that there is no measurable risk from consuming less than 1 oz AA per day. Others agree that no risks have been observed, but protest that safety has not been proven. Scientifically, only risk can be measured; the absence of risk (or absolute safety) can never be conclusively established. Given the present state of our knowledge, the question of whether or not light drinkers should be advised to abstain remains controversial among researchers and clinicians.

The ambiguity about how safe is safe and how healthy is healthy lends itself to the doubts that all parents experience when they plan a pregnancy. It is normal to hope for the ideal child who will be given every opportunity, and who will be as perfect as one can imagine. Following conception, parents are confronted with the uncertainty of multiple genetic and environmental risks. Risks can be minimized by avoiding established dangers, however they cannot be eliminated. Realistic parents must accept the limits of perfectibility. As pregnancy proceeds they must live with uncertainty but not with exaggerated fear and guilt.

There are hazards in exaggerating risk. The pregnant woman is confronted with many ordinary activities in her life which pose a small but identifiable risk. Although dangers from infectious diseases and starvation have diminished, we will never have a risk-free environment. Driving an automobile and breathing city air can be hazardous. While we hope to protect the fetus as completely as possible, in reality, risks begin at conception and are unavoidable. The total effect of excluding all risk would be so stifling that pregnancy would be like living in a greenhouse. The subsequent stress from the preoccupation with possible dangers may be a greater danger than any of the activities themselves. Pregnancy can be a burdensome time in which the mother may grow resentful of her child rather than developing positive maternal feelings. She cannot enjoy pregnancy when she is constrained by a multitude of prohibitions which may overwhelm her. The guilt, anxiety, and stress of an overly restricted lifestyle may cause neuroendocrine changes in the pregnant woman which can be harmful to the fetus. Stress-related elevation of ACTH and corticosterone has been associated experimentally with malformations (Stechler and Halton, 1983).

When the hazards of alcohol are exaggerated, light drinkers who have abnormal children are burdened with guilt and anxiety about their alcohol consumption, when, in fact, the problems were caused by any one of many environmental or genetic factors. Family conflicts arise when husbands accuse wives of causing their child's birth defects, and the interfamilial stresses can impede mother–infant bonding.

Women must be relieved, therefore, of the burden of believing that they can control all the factors that influence their babies' health. Distortion and exaggeration of the mother's role can cause unrealistic expectations for parenting. Although a mother's precautions during pregnancy contribute to the health of the fetus, she cannot guarantee it. Physicians should not foster an unrealistic illusion of control.

Misleading presentations of what is known about the causes of birth defects encourage women to believe that they are fully responsible for the health of their babies. The role of maternal drinking in the etiology of abnormalities is sometimes overstated. For example, Clarren and Smith (1978) stated, "Of the known causes of mental retardation, FAS is the third most common." The Third Special Report to Congress extended this statement to "FAS . . . (is) . . . the third leading cause of birth defects with associated mental retardation (HEW, 1978, p. 188). Others ʰave distorted it further and claimed, "Maternal alcohol consumption during gestation is a leading cause of mental deficiency in the Western world" (Sulik and Johnston, 1983, p. 257), and "Ingestion of alcohol by pregnant mothers is the third leading cause of mental retardation" (Altura et al, 1983). Many FAS programs have incorporated this statement in prevention campaigns. These last two statements are misleading. In fact, only 10% of the cases of mental retardation are of known origin; in 90% the causes are unknown. Clarren and Smith's statement, which actually asserts a connection between FAS and only 5% or less of the cases of mental retardation, has been misinterpreted as a claim about the total spectrum of retardation.

Unnecessary deprivation narrows the life of the pregnant woman. A woman should be given the opportunity to make informed choices based on current medical evidence. When a mother assumes the responsibility for determining a lifestyle and deciding which risks she is willing to tolerate, she gains a sense of mastering her own life and a sense of personal freedom. This reduces stress, improves her chances of having a happy and healthy pregnancy, and lessens resentment that her baby caused her to abandon her normal life activities.

With all the complexity, the clinician wonders if the possibility that some women can safely consume 1–2 drinks per day (never exceeding 1 oz AA) is worthy of consideration. We think it is, and that informed professionals can help each woman make her own decision. For the most cautious, abstention removes all danger from alcohol; there seems to be no harm from not drinking. However, the recommendation that all women should abstain from drinking during pregnancy is not based on scientific evidence, since no risks have been observed from consumption of small quantities. Issuing health recommendations which cannot be demonstrated as fact helps legitimize unproven, superstitious health fads. Furthermore, exaggerating the facts about alcohol and pregnancy blurs the real dangers of heavy drinking. It distracts health professionals from treating problem drinkers and deflects public health efforts from the target population in greatest need.

Summary

Stimulated by the clinical recognition of the FAS, knowledge about the biochemistry and pathophysiology of alcohol use during pregnancy has expanded rapidly. Development of effective programs for prevention followed the increased scientific understanding. Although mass media campaigns have heightened public awareness, they have failed to change the behavior of pregnant women who drink heavily. These women, whose children are at serious risk, require individual supportive counselling. This can be effectively provided within the current health care delivery system. All professionals must assume responsibility for identifying and treating pregnant women abusing alcohol.

History and sociology document that the danger to the fetus from heavy drinking during pregnancy was once medically recognized but subsequently rejected when scientific findings were promulgated in an exaggerated and moralistic manner. Now that the early understanding of alcohol's effects on the fetus has become more extensive, repetition of this historical cycle must be avoided. Our total body of knowledge must be integrated, and further research must be undertaken to untangle the interacting metabolic, environmental, and social variables. Incorporating existing information into clinical practice will strengthen the effectiveness of prenatal health programs.

REFERENCES

Aase, JM: The fetal alcohol syndrome in American Indians: A high risk group. *Neurobehav Toxicol Teratol* 3:153–156, 1981.

Abel, EL: Effects of ethanol on pregnant rats and their offspring. *Psychopharmacology* 57:5–11, 1978.

Abel, EL: Prenatal effects of alcohol on adult learning in rat. *Pharmacol Biochem Behav* 10:239–243, 1979a.

Abel, EL: Effects of ethanol exposure during different gestation weeks of pregnancy on maternal weight gain and intrauterine growth retardation in the rat. *Neurobehav Toxicol* 1:145–151, 1979b.

Abel, EL: The fetal alcohol syndrome: behavioral teratology. *Psychol Bull* 87:29–50, 1980a.

Abel, EL: Procedural considerations in evaluating prenatal effects of alcohol in animals. *Neurobehav Toxicol* 2:167–174, 1980b.

Abel, EL: Prenatal exposure to beer, wine, whiskey, and ethanol: effects on postnatal growth and food and water consumption. *Neurobehav Toxicol Teratol* 3:49–51, 1981a.

Abel, EL: A critical evaluation of the obstetric use of alcohol in preterm labor. *Drug Alcohol Depend* 7:367–378, 1981b.

Abel, EL: Consumption of alcohol during pregnancy: a review of effects on growth and development of offspring. *Human Biology* 54:421–453, 1982a.

Abel, EL: Introduction. *Fetal Alcohol Syndrome,* Vol. II. CRC Press, Boca Raton, 1982b.

Abel, EL, Dintcheff, BA: Effects of prenatal alcohol exposure on growth and development in rats. *J Pharmacol Exp Ther* 207:916–921, 1978.

Abel, EL, Dintcheff, BA, Day, N: Effects of in utero exposure to alcohol, nicotine, and alcohol plus nicotine, on growth and development in rats. *Neurobehav Toxicol* 1:153–159, 1979.

Abel, EL, Greizerstein, HB: Ethanol-induced prenatal growth deficiency: changes in fetal body composition. *J Pharmacol Exp Ther* 211:668–671, 1979.

Abel, EL, Greizerstein, HB: Growth and development in animals prenatally exposed to alcohol. In EL Abel, ed, *Fetal Alcohol Syndrome*, Vol III, CRC Press, Boca Raton, 1982, pp 39–58.

Abel, EL, York, JL: Absence of effect of prenatal ethanol on adult emotionality and ethanol consumption in rats. *J Stud Alcohol* 40:547–553, 1979.

Agarwal, DP, Harada, S, Goedde, HW: Racial differences in biological sensitivity to ethanol: the role of alcohol dehydrogenase and aldehyde dehydrogenase isozymes. *Alcoholism Clin Exp Res* 5:12–16, 1981.

Aherne, W, Dunnill, MS: Morphometry of the human placenta. *Br Med Bull* 22:5–8, 1966.

Åkesson, C: Autoradiographic studies on the distribution of ^{14}C-2-ethanol and its non-volatile metabolites in the pregnant mouse. *Arch Int Pharmacodyn* 209:296–304, 1974.

Alcohol and spontaneous abortion (editorial). *Lancet* 2:188, 1980.

Alpert, JJ, Day, N, Dooling, E, Hingson, R, Oppenheimer, E, Rosett, HL, Weiner, L, Zuckerman B: Maternal alcohol consumption and newborn assessment: methodology of the Boston City Hospital prospective study. *Neurobehav Toxicol Teratol* 3:195–201, 1981.

Altshuler, HL, Amirian, JH: The fetal alcohol syndrome in rhesus monkeys. I. Development of the model. *Teratology* (in press).

Altshuler, HL, Shippenberg, TS: A subhuman primate model for fetal alcohol syndrome research. *Neurobehav Toxicol Teratol* 3:121–126, 1981.

Altura, BM, Altura, BT, Carella, A, Chatterjee, M, Halevy, S, Tejani, N: Alcohol produces spasms of human umbilical blood vessels: relationship to fetal alcohol syndrome (FAS). *Eur J Pharmacol* 86:311–312, 1983.

Amankwah, KS, Weberg, AD, Kaufmann, RC: Ultrastructural changes in preputial neural tissues: effects of maternal drinking. *Early Hum Dev* 6:375–380, 1982.

American Council on Science and Health: Alcohol Use During Pregnancy. Summit, New Jersey, 1981.

American Medical Association, Council on Scientific Affairs: Fetal effects of maternal alcohol use. *J Am Med Assoc* 249:2517–2521, 1983.

Anand, S, Van Thiel, DH: Prenatal and neonatal exposure to cimetidine results in gonadal and sexual dysfunction in adult males. *Science* 218:493–494, 1982.

Anders, K, Persaud, TVN: Compensatory embryonic development in the rat following maternal treatment with ethanol. *Anat Anaz* 148:375–383, 1980.

Anderson, RA: Endocrine balance as a factor in the etiology of the fetal alcohol syndrome. *Neurobehav Toxicol Teratol* 3:89–104, 1981.

Anderson, RA, Beyler, SA, Zaneveld, LJD: Alterations of male reproduction induced by chronic ingestion of ethanol: Development of an animal model. *Fert Steril* 30:103–105, 1978.

Anderson, WJ, Sides, GR: Alcohol-induced defects in cerebellar development in the rat. In M Galanter, ed, *Currents in Alcoholism,* Vol 5. Grune and Stratton, New York, 1978, pp 135–153.

Badr, FM, Badr, RS: Induction of dominant lethal mutation in male mice by ethyl alcohol. *Nature* 253:134–136, 1975.

Bannigan, J, Burke, P: Ethanol teratogenicity in mice: a light microscopic study. *Teratology* 26:247–254, 1982.

Barden, TP, Peter, JB, Merkatz, IR: Ritodrine hydrochloride: a betamimetic agent for use in preterm labor. I. Pharmacology, clinical history, administration, side effects, and safety. *Obstet Gynecol* 56:1–6, 1980.

Barrison, IG, Wright, JT, Sampson, B, Morris, NF, Murray-Lyon, IM: Screening for alcohol abuse in pregnancy. *Br Med J* 285:1318, 1982.

Bauer-Moffett, C, Altman, J: Ethanol-induced reductions in cerebellar growth of infant rats. *Exp Neurol* 48:378–382, 1975.

Bauer-Moffett, C, Altman, J: The effect of ethanol chronically administered to preweanling rats on cerebellar development: a morphological study. *Brain Res* 114:249–268, 1977.

Becker, H, Zaunschirm, H, Muntean, W, Domej, W: Alkoholembryopathie und maligner tumor. *Wiener Klinische Wochenschrift* 94:364–365, 1982.

Beecher, L: *Six Sermons on the Nature, Occasions, Signs, Evils, and Remedy of Intemperance.* Boston, Crocker and Brewster, 1827.

Bennett, AL, Sorette, MP, Greenwood, MRC: Effect of chronic paternal ethanol consumption on 19-day rat fetuses. *Fed Proc* 41:71, 1982.

Berkowitz, GS: An epidemiologic study of preterm delivery. *Am J Epidemiol* 113:81–92, 1981.

Berkowitz, GS, Holford, TR, Berkowitz, RL: Effects of cigarette smoking, alcohol, coffee and tea consumption on preterm delivery. *Early Hum Dev* 7:239–250, 1982.

Bierich, JR: Pränatale schädigungen durch alkohol (Prenatal damage from alcohol). *Der Internist* 19:131–139, 1978.

Bierich, J, Majewski, F, Michaelis, R, Tillner, I: Das embryofetale alkoholsyndrom (Embryofetal alcohol syndrome). *Eur J Pediatr* 121:155–177, 1976.

Binkiewicz, A, Robinson, MJ, Senior, B: Pseudo-Cushing syndrome caused by alcohol in breast milk. *J Pediatr* 93:965–967, 1978.

Blomstrand, R: Observations on the formation of ethanol in the intestinal tract in man. *Life Sci* 10:575–582, 1971.

Boggan, WO, Randall, CL, Dodds, HM: Delayed sexual maturation in female C57BL/6J mice prenatally exposed to alcohol. *Res Commun Chem Pathol Pharmacol* 23:117–125, 1979.

Bohman, M, Sigvardsson, S, Cloninger, CR: Maternal inheritance of alcohol abuse: cross-fostering analysis of adopted women. *Arch Gen Psych* 38:965–969, 1981.

Bond, NW: Prenatal alcohol exposure in rodents: A review of its effects on offspring activity and learning ability. *Australian J Psychol* 33: 331–344, 1981.

Bond, NW, DiGiusto, EL: Effects of prenatal alcohol consumption on open-field behavior and alcohol preference in rats. *Psychopharmacology* 46:163–165, 1976.

Bond, NW, DiGiusto, EL: Prenatal alcohol consumption and open-field behavior in rats: Effects of age at time of testing. *Psychopharmacology* 52:311–312, 1977.

Borges, S, Lewis, PD: A study of alcohol effects on the brain during gestation and lactation. *Teratology* 25:283–289, 1982.

Borges, S, Lewis, PD: The effect of ethanol on the cellular composition of the cerebellum. *Neuropathol Appl Neurobiol* 9:53–60, 1983.

Bottoms, SF, Judge, NE, Kuhnert, PM, Sokol, RJ: Thiocyanate and drinking during pregnancy. *Alcoholism Clin Exp Res* 6:391–395, 1982.

Brandt, EN: Alcohol consumption during pregnancy. Testimony before the Subcommittee on Alcoholism and Drug Abuse of the Committee on Labor and Human Resources, US Senate, Washington, DC, US Government Printing Office, September 21, 1982, pp 9–23.

Brazelton, TB: Neonatal Behavioral Assessment Scale. Lippincott, Philadelphia, 1973.

Brown, NA, Goulding, EH, Fabro, S: Ethanol embryotoxicity: direct effects on mammalian embryos in vitro. *Science* 206:573–575, 1979.

Burton, R: *The Anatomy of Melancholy.* Vol 1, Part I, Section 2: Causes of melancholy. William Tegg, London, 1906 [Orig. 1621].

Cahalan, D, Cissin, IR, Crossley, HM: *American Drinking Practices,* New Brunswick, New Jersey, Rutgers Center of Alcohol Studies, 1969.

Campbell, MA, Fantel, AG: Teratogenicity of acetaldehyde in vitro: relevance to the fetal alcohol syndrome. *Life Sci* 32:2641-2647, 1983.

Caritis, SN, Edelstone, DI, Mueller-Heubach, E: Pharmacologic inhibition of preterm labor. *Am J Obstet Gynecol* 133:557–578, 1979.

Casey, PH: Environment, genes, and alcohol (letter). *Pediatrics* 71:989, 1983.

Castells, S, Mark, E, Abaci, F, Schwartz, E: Growth retardation in fetal alcohol syndrome: unresponsiveness to growth-promoting hormones. *Dev Pharmacol Ther* 3:232–241, 1981.

Cavdar, AO: DiGeorges syndrome and fetal alcohol syndrome (letter). *Am J Dis Child* 137:806–807, 1983.

Chafetz, ME, Blane, HT, Hill, MJ: Children of alcoholics: observations in a child guidance clinic. *Quart J Stud Alc 32*:687–698, 1971.

Chappel, JN, Schnoll, SH: Doctors' attitudes: effect on the treatment of chemically dependent patients. *J Am Med Assoc 239*:2318–2319, 1977.

Chasnoff, IJ, Diggs, G, Schnoll, SH: Fetal alcohol effects and maternal cough syrup abuse. *Am J Dis Child 135*:968, 1981.

Chen, J-S, Driscoll, CD, Riley, EP: Ontogeny of suckling behavior in rats prenatally exposed to alcohol. *Teratology 26*:145–153, 1982.

Cheng, Y-S: Pregnancy in liver cirrhosis and/or portal hypertension. *Am J Obstet Gynecol 128*:812–822, 1977.

Chernick, V, Childiaeva R, Ioffe, S: Effects of maternal alcohol intake and smoking on neonatal EEG and anthropometric measurements. *Am J Obstet Gynecol 146*:41–47, 1983.

Chernoff, GF: The fetal alcohol syndrome in mice: an animal model. *Teratology 15*:223–230, 1977.

Chernoff, GF: The fetal alcohol syndrome in mice: maternal variables. *Teratology 22*:71–75, 1980.

Chin, JH, Goldstein, DB, Parsons, LM: Fluidity and lipid composition of mouse biomembranes during adaptation to ethanol. *Alcoholism Clin Exp Res 3*:47–49, 1979.

Christiaens, L, Mizon, JP, Delmarie, G: Sur la descendance des alcooliques (On the offspring of alcoholics). *Ann Pediatr (Paris) 36*:257–262, 1960.

Christoffel, KK, Salafsky, I: Fetal alcohol syndrome in dizygotic twins. *J Pediatr 87*:963–967, 1975.

Church, MW, Holloway, JA: Postnatal development of brainstem evoked potentials in rat pups prenatally exposed to ethanol: a preliminary report. *Alcohol Tech Rept 9*:7–12, 1980.

Cicero, TJ: Sex differences in the effects of alcohol and other psychoactive drugs on endocrine function: clinical and experimental evidence. In OJ Kalant, ed, *Alcohol and Drug Problems in Women,* Plenum Press, New York, 1980, pp. 545–593.

Clarren, SK: Recognition of fetal alcohol syndrome. *J Am Med Assoc 245*:2436–2439, 1981.

Clarren, SK: The diagnosis and treatment of fetal alcohol syndrome. *Pediatrics 8*:41–46, 1982.

Clarren, SK, Alvord, EC Jr, Sumi, SM, Streissguth, AP, Smith, DW: Brain malformations related to prenatal exposure to ethanol. *J Pediatr 92*:64–67, 1978.

Clarren, SK, Bowden, DM: Fetal alcohol syndrome: a new primate model for binge drinking and its relevance to human ethanol teratogenesis. *J Pediatr 101*:819–824, 1982.

Clarren, SK, Smith, DW: The fetal alcohol syndrome. *N Engl J Med* 298:1063–1067, 1978.

Coffey, TG: Beer Street: Gin Lane: Some views of 18th century drinking. *Quart J Stud Alc* 27:669–692, 1966.

Cohen, J, Cohen, P: *Applied Multiple Regression/Correlation Analysis for the Behavioral Sciences.* J Wiley & Sons, New York, 1975.

Cook, LN, Shott, RJ, Andrews, BF: Acute transplacental ethanol intoxication. *Am J Dis Child* 129:1075–1076, 1975.

Cooperman, MT, Davidoff, F, Spark, R, Pallotta, J: Clinical studies of alcoholic ketoacidosis. *Diabetes* 23:433–439, 1974.

Cork, M: *The Forgotten Children: A Study of Children with Alcoholic Parents.* Alcoholism and Drug Addiction Research Foundation, Toronto, 1969.

Cremin, BJ, Jaffer, Z: Radiologic aspects of the fetal alcohol syndrome. *Pediatr Radiol* 11:151–153, 1981.

Crépin, G, Querleu, D, Bigant, C, Delahousse, G, Decocq, J, Delcroix, M, Caquant, F: Cirrhose hépatique et grossesse: A propos de cinq observations (Cirrhosis of the liver and pregnancy: a review of five case histories). *Med Chirurg Dig* 6:127–135, 1977.

Davies, DL, Smith, DE: A Golgi study of mouse hippocampal CA1 pyramidal neurons following perinatal ethanol exposure. *Neurosci Lett* 26:49–54, 1981.

DeBeukelaer, MM, Randall, CL, Stroud, DR: Renal anomalies in the fetal alcohol syndrome. *J Pediatr* 91:759–760, 1977.

DeElejalde, F: Inadequate mothering: patterns and treatment. *Bull Menninger Clinic* 35:182–198, 1971.

Dehaene, P, Crepin, G, Delahousse, G, Querleu, D, Walbaum, R, Titran, M, Samaille-Villette, C: Aspects épidémiologiques du syndrome d'alcoolisme foetal. *Nouv Presse Med* 10:2639–2643, 1981.

Dehaene, P, Samaille-Villette, C, Samaille, P-P, Crépin, G, Walbaum, R, Deroubaix, P, Blanc-Garin, A-P: Le syndrome d'alcoolisme foetal dans le Nord de la France (Fetal alcohol syndrome in the north of France). *Rev l'Alcoolisme,* 23:145–158, 1977a.

Dehaene, P, Walbaum, R, Titran, M, Samaille-Villette, C, Samaille, P, Crépin, G, Delahousse, G, Decocq, J, Delcroix, M, Caquant, F, Querleu, D: La descendance des mères alcooliques chroniques: a propos de 16 cas d'alcoolisme foetal (The offspring of alcoholic mothers: a report of 16 cases of fetal alcohol syndrome). *Rev Francaise Gynécol d'Obstétrique* 72:491–498, 1977b.

Deitrich, RA, Petersen, DR: Interaction of ethanol with other drugs. In E Majchrowicz and EP Noble, eds, *Biochemistry and Pharmacology of Ethanol,* Vol II. Plenum Press, New York, 1979, pp. 283–302.

Detering, N, Collins, RM, Jr, Hawkins, RL, Ozand, PT, Karahasan, A:

Comparative effects of ethanol and malnutrition on the development of catecholamine neurons: Changes in neurotransmitter levels. *J Neurochem* 34:1587–1593, 1980a.

Detering, N, Collins, RM, Jr, Hawkins, RL, Ozand, PT, Karahasan, A: Comparative effect of ethanol and malnutrition on the development of catecholamine neurons: changes in norepinephrine turnover. *J Neurochem* 34:1788–1791, 1980b.

Detering, N, Edwards, E, Ozand, P, Karahasan, A: Comparative effects of ethanol and malnutrition on the development of catecholamine neurons: changes in specific activities of enzymes. *J Neurochem* 39:297–304, 1980c.

Detering, N, Reed, WD, Ozand, PT, Karahasan, A: The effects of maternal ethanol consumption in the rat on the development of their offspring. *J Nutr* 109:999–1009, 1979.

Dexter, JD, Tumbleson, ME, Decker, JD, Middleton, CC: Fetal alcohol syndrome in sinclair (S-1) miniature swine. *Alcoholism Clin Exp Res* 4:146–151, 1980.

Dexter, JD, Tumbleson, ME, Decker, JD, Middleton, CC: Comparison of the offspring of three serial pregnancies during voluntary alcohol consumption in Sinclair (S-1) miniature swine. *Neurobehav Toxicol Teratol* 5:229–231, 1983.

Diamond, S: *Information and Error*. Basic Books, New York, 1959, p. 82.

Diaz, J, Samson, HH: Impaired brain growth in neonatal rats exposed to ethanol. *Science* 208:751–753, 1980.

Dobbing, J: The later growth of the brain and its vulnerability. *Pediatrics* 53:2–6, 1974.

Dreosti, IE, Ballard, FJ, Belling, GB, Record, IR, Manuel, SJ, Hetzel, BS: The effect of ethanol and acetaldehyde on DNA synthesis in growing cells and on fetal development in the rat. *Alcoholism Clin Exp Res* 5:357–362, 1981.

Drillien, CM: *The Growth and Development of the Prematurely Born Infant*. Livingstone, Edinburgh, 1964.

Driscoll, CD, Chen, JS, Riley, EP: Operant DRL performance in rats following prenatal alcohol exposure. *Neurobehav Toxicol* 2:207–211, 1980.

Druse, MJ, Hofteig, JH: The effect of chronic maternal alcohol consumption on the development of central nervous system myelin subfractions in rat offspring. *Drug Alcohol Depend* 2:421–429, 1977.

Druse, MJ, Waddell, CS, and Haas, RG: Maternal ethanol consumption during the third trimester of pregnancy: synaptic plasma membrane glycoproteins and gangliosides in offspring. *Substance and Alcohol Actions/Misuse* 2:359–368, 1981.

Dubowitz, L, Dubowitz, A, Goldberg, C: Clinical assessment of gestational age in the newborn infant. *J Pediatr* 77:1–10, 1970.

Dunigan, TH, Werlin, SL: Extrahepatic biliary atresia and renal anomalies in fetal alcohol syndrome. *Am J Dis Child 135*:1067–1068, 1981.

Dupuis, C, Dehaene, P, Deroubaix-Tella, P, Blanc-Garin, AP, Rey, C, Carpentier-Couralt, C: Les cardiopathies des enfants nés de mère alcoolique (Cardiopathy in children born of alcoholic mothers). *Arch Maladies Coeur Vaisseaux 71*:565–572, 1978.

Edwards, J: *The Temperance Manual.* New York, American Tract Society, 1847.

Ehrhardt, AA, Meyer-Bahlburg, HFL: Prenatal sex hormones and the developing brain: effects on psychosexual differentiation and cognitive function. *Ann Rev Med 30*:417–430, 1979.

El-Guebaly, N, Offord, DR: The offspring of alcoholics: critical review. *Am J Psychiatry 134*:357–365, 1977.

Ellis, FW, Pick, JR: An animal model of the fetal alcohol syndrome in beagles. *Alcoholism Clin Exp Res 4*:123–134, 1980.

English, D, Bower, C: Alcohol consumption, pregnancy, and low birthweight (letter). *Lancet 1*:1111, 1983.

Fabro, S: Alcoholic beverage consumption and outcome of pregnancy. In *The Fetal Alcohol Syndrome—Public Awareness Campaign,* Department of the Treasury, February 1979, pp. 37–199.

Fabro, S: In utero alcohol exposure: threshold for effects? A Medical Letter *Repro Toxicol 1*:11–14, 1982.

Farber, JM: Letter. *Pediatrics 70*:323–324, 1982.

Ferreira, AJ: The pregnant mother's emotional attitude and its reflection upon the newborn. *Am J Orthopsychiat 30*:553–561, 1960.

Finkelstein, N, Brown, KN, Laham, CQ: Alcoholic mothers and guilt: issues for caregivers. *Alcohol Health Res World 4*:45–51, 1981.

Finnegan, LP, ed: Drug Dependence in Pregnancy: Clinical Management of Mother and Child. USDHEW, 1979, pp. 63–82.

Finnegan, LP, Fehr, KO: The effects of opiates, sedative-hypnotics, amphetamines, cannabis, and other psychoactive drugs on the fetus and newborn. In OJ Kalant, ed, *Alcohol and Drug Problems in Women,* Plenum Press, New York, 1980, pp. 653–723.

Finucane, BT: Difficult intubation associated with the foetal alcohol syndrome. *Canad Anaesth Soc J 27*:574–575, 1980.

Fisher, SE, Atkinson, M, Burnap, JK, Jacobson, S, Sehgal, PK, Scott, W, Van Thiel, DV: Ethanol-associated selective fetal malnutrition: a contributing factor in the fetal alcohol syndrome. *Alcoholism Clin Exp Res 6*:197–201, 1982.

Fisher, SE, Atkinson, M, Van Thiel, DH, Rosenblum, E, David, R, Holzman, I: Selective fetal malnutrition: the effect of ethanol and acetaldehyde upon in vitro uptake of alpha amino isobutyric acid by human placenta. *Life Sci 20*:1283–1288, 1981.

Fitze, F, Spahr, A, Pescia, G: Familienstudie zum Problem des Embryo-fötalen Alkoholsyndroms (Embryofetal alcohol syndrome: followup of a family). *Schweizerische Rundschau für Medizin (Praxis)* 67:1338–1354, 1978.

Fitzgerald, JL, Mulford, HA: Distribution of alcohol consumption and problem drinking: Comparison of sales records and survey data. *J Stud Alcohol* 39:879–893, 1978.

Flink, EB: Mineral metabolism in alcoholism. In B Kissin and H Begleiter, eds, *The Biology of Alcoholism, Vol I. Biochemistry.* Plenum, New York, 1971, pp. 377–395.

Flint, EF: Severe childhood deafness in Glasgow, 1965–1979. *J Laryngol Otology* 97:421–425, 1983.

Flynn, A, Martier, SS, Sokol, RJ, Miller, SI, Golden, NL, Del Villano, BC: Zinc status of pregnant alcoholic women: a determinant of fetal outcome. *Lancet* 1:572–574, 1981.

Fox, HE, Steinbrecher, M, Pessel, D, Inglis, J, Medvid, L, Angel, E: Maternal ethanol ingestion and the occurrence of human fetal breathing movements. *Am J Obstet Gynecol* 132:354–358, 1978.

Frias, JL, Wilson, AL, King, GJ: A cephalometric study of fetal alcohol syndrome. *J Pediatr* 101:870–873, 1982.

Fried, PA: Marijuana use by pregnant women: neurobehavioral effects in neonates. *Drug Alcohol Depend* 6:415–424, 1980.

Fried, PA: Marijuana use by pregnant women and effects on offspring: an update. *Neurobehav Toxicol Teratol* 4:451–454, 1982.

Fried, PA, Watkinson, B, Grant, A, Knights, RM: Changing patterns of soft drug use prior to and during pregnancy: a prospective study. *Drug Alcohol Depend* 6:323–343, 1980.

Fuchs, F, Fuchs, AR, Poblete, VF, Jr, Risk, A: Effect of alcohol on threatened premature labor. *Am J Obstet Gynecol* 99:627–637, 1967.

Garber, JM: Corneal curvature in the fetal alcohol syndrome: preliminary report. *J Am Optomol Assoc* 53:641–644, 1982.

George, MD: London Life in the Eighteenth Century. Capricorn, New York, 1965.

Ghishan, FK, Henderson, G, Meneely, R: Intestinal function in infant rats: effect of maternal chronic ethanol ingestion. *J Nutr* 111:1124–1127, 1981.

Ghishan, FK, Patwardhan, R, Greene, HL: Fetal alcohol syndrome: inhibition of placental zinc transport as a potential mechanism for fetal growth retardation in the rat. *J Lab Clin Med* 100:45–52, 1982.

Gibson, GT, Baghurst, PA, Colley, DP: Maternal alcohol, tobacco and cannabis consumption and the outcome of pregnancy. *Aust N Z J Obstet Gynaecol* 23:15–19, 1983.

Giknis, MLA, Damjanov, I, Rubin, E: The differential transplacental effects of ethanol in four mouse strains. *Neurobehav Toxicol 2*: 235–237, 1980.

Gilbert, RM: Caffeine as a drug of abuse. In RJ Gibbins, Y Israel, H Kalant, RE Popham, W Schmidt, and RG Smart, eds, *Research Advances in Alcohol and Drug Problems*, Vol 3, Wiley, New York, 1976, pp. 49–176.

Goetzman, BW, Kagan, J, Blankenship, WI: Expansion of the fetal alcohol syndrome. *Clin Res 23*:100A, 1975.

Golden, NL, Sokol, RJ, Kuhnert, BR, Bottoms, S: Maternal alcohol use and infant development. *Pediatrics 70*:931–934, 1982.

Goldstein, G, Arulanantham, K: Neural tube defect and renal anomalies in a child with fetal alcohol syndrome. *J Pediatr 93*:636–637, 1978.

Goodwin, DW: Is alcoholism hereditary? A review and critique. *Arch Gen Psychiatry 25*:545–549, 1971.

Goodwin, DW, Schulsinger, F, Hermansen, L, Guze, SB, Winokur, G: Alcohol problems in adoptees raised apart from alcoholic biological parents. *Arch Gen Psychiatry 28*:238–243, 1973.

Goujard, J, Kaminski, M, Rumeau-Rouquette, C, Schwartz, D: Maternal smoking, alcohol consumption, and abruptio placentae. *Am J Obstet Gynecol 130*:738–739, 1978.

Greenhouse, BS, Hook, R, Hehre, FW: Aspiration pneumonia following intravenous administration of alcohol during labor. *J Am Med Assoc 210*:2393–2395, 1969.

Greenland, S, Staisch, KJ, Brown, N, Gross, SJ: Effects of marijuana on human pregnancy, labor, and delivery. *Neurobehav Toxicol Teratol 4*:447–450, 1982.

Grundfast, KM: The role of the audiologist and otologist in the identification of the dysmorphic child. *Ear and Hearing 4*:24–30, 1983.

Habbick, BF, Casey, R, Zaleski, WA, Murphy, F: Liver abnormalities in three patients with fetal alcohol syndrome. *Lancet 1*:580–581, 1979.

Haggard, HW, Jellinek, EM: *Alcohol Explored*. Doubleday, Garden City, 1942.

Halkka, O, Eriksson, K: The effects of chronic ethanol consumption on goniomitosis in the rat. In MM Gross, ed, *Alcohol Intoxication and Withdrawal: Experimental Studies*, Vol 3, Plenum, New York, 1977, pp. 1–6.

Hanson, JW, Jones, KL, Smith, DW: Fetal alcohol syndrome: experience with 41 patients. *J Am Med Assoc 235*:1458–1460, 1976.

Hanson, JW, Streissguth, AP, Smith, DW: The effects of moderate alcohol consumption during pregnancy on fetal growth and morphogenesis. *J Pediatr 92*:457–460, 1978.

Harlap, S, Shiono, PH: Alcohol, smoking and incidence of spontaneous abortions in the first and second trimester. *Lancet* 2:173–176, 1980.

Havers, W, Majewski, F, Olbing, H, and Eikenberg, H-U: Anomalies of the kidneys and genitourinary tract in alcohol embryopathy. *J Urology* 124:108–110, 1980.

Havlicek, V, Childiaeva, R: Sleep EEG in newborns of mothers using alcohol. In EL Abel, ed, *Fetal Alcohol Syndrome,* Vol II, CRC Press, Boca Raton, 1982, pp. 149–178.

Hayden, MR, Nelson, MM: The fetal alcohol syndrome. *S Afr Med J* 54:571–574, 1978.

Henderson, GI, Hoyumpa, AM, Jr, McClain, C, Schenker, S: The effects of chronic and acute alcohol administration on fetal development in the rat. *Alcoholism Clin Exp Res* 3:99–106, 1979.

Henderson, GI, Hoyumpa, AM, Jr, Rothschild, MA, Schenker, S: Effect of ethanol and ethanol-induced hypothermia on protein synthesis in pregnant and fetal rats. *Alcoholism Clin Exp Res* 4:165–177, 1980.

Henderson, GI, Turner, D, Patwhardan, RV, Lumeng, L, Hoyumpa, AM, Jr, Schenker, S: Inhibition of placental valine uptake after acute and chronic maternal ethanol consumption. *J Pharmacol Exp Ther* 216:465–472, 1981.

Herrmann, J, Pallister, PD, Optiz, JM: Tetraectrodactyly and other skeletal manifestations in the fetal alcohol syndrome. *Eur J Pediatr* 133:221–226, 1980.

Heuyer, O, Misès, R, Dereux, J-F: La descendances des alcooliques (Offspring of alcoholics). *Presse Med* 65:657–658, 1957.

Hill, RM: Drugs ingested by pregnant women. *Clin Pharmacol Ther 14:* 654–659, 1973.

Hill, RM: Fetal malformations and antiepileptic drugs. *Am J Dis Child* 130:923–925, 1976.

Hill, RM: Adverse effects of prenatal drug therapy. In BL Mirkin, ed, *Clinical Pharmacology,* Year Book Medical Publishers, Inc., Chicago, 1978, pp. 199–219.

Hingson, R, Alpert, JJ, Day, N, Dooling, E, Kayne, H, Morelock, S, Oppenheimer, E, Zuckerman, B: Effects of maternal drinking and marijuana use on fetal growth and development. *Pediatrics 70:* 539–546, 1982.

Ho, BT, Fritchie, GE, Idänpään-Heikkilä, JE, McIsaac, WM: Placental transfer and tissue distribution of ethanol-1-^{14}C: a radioautographic study in monkeys and hamsters. *Quart J Study Alc* 33:485–493, 1972.

Hoberman, HD: Adduct formation between hemoglobin and 5-Deoxy-Dxylulose-1-phosphate. *Biochem Biophys Res Commun* 90:764–768, 1979.

Hoberman, HD, Chiodo, SM: Elevation of the hemoglobin A1 fraction in alcoholism. *Alcoholism Clin Exp Res* 6:260–266, 1982.

Hofteig, JH, Druse, MJ: Central nervous system myelination in rats exposed to ethanol in utero. *Drug Alcohol Depend* 3:429–434, 1978.

Holmberg, PC: Central-nervous-system defects in children born to mothers exposed to organic solvents during pregnancy. *Lancet* 2: 177–179, 1979.

Horiguchi, T, Suzuki, K, Comas-Urrutia, AC, Mueller-Heubach, E, Boyer-Milic, AM, Baratz, RA, Morishima, HO, James, LS, Adamsons, K: Effect of ethanol upon uterine activity and fetal acid-base state of the rhesus monkey. *Am J Obstet Gynecol* 109:910–917, 1975.

Hornstein, L, Crowe, C, Gruppo, R: Adrenal carcinoma in child with history of fetal alcohol syndrome. *Lancet* 2:1292–1293, 1977.

Horrobin, DF: A biochemical basis for alcoholism and alcohol-induced damage including the fetal alcohol syndrome and cirrhosis: Interference with essential fatty acid and prostaglandin metabolism. *Med Hypotheses* 6:929–942, 1980.

Hrbek, A, Iversen, K, Olsson, T: Evaluation of cerebral function in newborn infants with fetal growth retardation. In J Courjon, F Mauguiere, M Revol, eds, *Clinical Applications of Evoked Potentials in Neurology*. Raven Press, New York, 1982, pp. 89–95.

Hrbek, A, Karlberg, P, Kjellmer, I, Torsten, O, Riha, M: Clinical application of evoked electroencephalographic responses in newborn infants I: perinatal asphyxia. *Dev Med Child Neurol* 19:34–44, 1977.

Hurley, LS: The fetal alcohol syndrome: possible implications of nutrient deficiencies. In TK Li, S Schenker, L Lumeng, eds, *Alcohol and Nutrition*, Res Mon #2, NIAAA, Washington D.C., 1979, pp. 367–379.

Idänpään-Heikkilä, J, Jouppila, P, Akerblom, HK, Isoaho, R, Kauppila, E, Koivisto, M: Elimination and metabolic effects of ethanol in mother, fetus and newborn infant. *Am J Obstet Gynecol* 112:387–393, 1972.

Ijaiya, K, Schwenk, A, Gladtke, E: Fetales alkoholsyndrom (Fetal alcohol syndrome). *Dtsch Med Wochenschr* 101:1563–1568, 1976.

Iosub, S, Fuchs, M, Bingol, N, Gromisch, DS: Fetal alcohol syndrome revisited. *Pediatrics* 68:475–479, 1981.

Jackson, JK: The adjustment of the family to the crisis of alcoholism. *Quart J Stud Alc* 15:562–586, 1954.

Jacobson, S, Rich, J, Tovsky, NJ: Delayed myelination and lamination in the cerebral cortex of the albino rat as a result of the fetal alcohol syndrome. In: M Galanter, ed, *Currents in Alcoholism,* Vol 5, Grune and Stratton, New York, 1978, pp. 123–133.

Jaffer, Z, Nelson, M, Beighton, P: Bone fusion in the foetal alcohol syndrome. *J Bone Jt Surg (Br)* 63B:569–571, 1981.

Janz, D: The teratogenic risk of antiepileptic drugs. *Epilepsia* 16:159–169, 1975.

Jellinek, EM: *The Disease Concept of Alcoholism,* New College University Press, New Haven, 1960, pp. 36–40.

Jenkins, DW, Eckle, RE, Craig, JW: Alcoholic ketoacidosis. *J Am Med Assoc* 217:177–183, 1971.

Joffe, JM: Alcohol and pregnancy (Letter). *Science* 221:1244–1246, 1983.

Joffe, JM, Soyka, LF: Paternal drug exposure: effects on reproduction and progeny. *Seminars in Perinatology* 6:116–124, 1982.

Johnson, KG: Fetal alcohol syndrome. *Rocky Mt Med J* 76:64–65, 1979.

Johnson, S, Knight, R, Marmer, D, Steele, RW: Immune deficiency in fetal alcohol syndrome. *Pediatr Res* 15:908–911, 1981.

Jones, BM, Jones, MK: Women and alcohol: intoxication, metabolism and the menstrual cycle. In M Greenblatt and MA Schuckit, eds, *Alcoholism Problems in Women and Children,* Grune and Stratton, New York, 1976, pp. 103–136.

Jones, KL, Hanson, JW, Smith, DW: Palpebral fissure size in newborn infants. *J Pediatr* 92:787, 1978.

Jones, KL, Smith, DW: Recognition of the fetal alcohol syndrome in early infancy. *Lancet* 2:999–1001, 1973.

Jones, KL, Smith, DW, Streissguth, AP, Myrianthopoulos, NC: Outcome of offspring of chronic alcoholic women. *Lancet* 1:1076–1078, 1974.

Jones, KL, Smith, DW, Ulleland, CN, Streissguth, AP: Pattern of malformation in offspring of chronic alcoholic mothers. *Lancet* 1:1267–1271, 1973.

Jones, PJH, Leichter, J, Lee, M: Uptake of zinc, folate and analogs of glucose and amino acid by the rat fetus exposed to alcohol in utero. *Nutrition Rept Int* 24:75–83, 1981.

Jones, RW, Helrich, AR: Treatment of alcoholism by physicians in private practice: a national survey. *Quart J Stud Alc* 33:117–131, 1972.

Kakihana, R, Butte, JC, Moore, JA: Endocrine effects of maternal alcoholization: plasma and brain testosterone, dihydrotestosterone, estradiol, and corticosterone. *Alcoholism Clin Exp Res* 4:57–61, 1980.

Kalter, H, Warkany, J: Congenital malformations (Part I): etiologic factors and their role in prevention. *N Engl J Med* 308:424–431, 1983a.

Kalter, H, Warkany, J: Congenital malformations (Part II). *N Engl J Med* 308:491–497, 1983b.

Kaminski, M, Franc, M, Lebouvier, M, duMazaubrun, C, Rumeau-Rouquette, C: Moderate alcohol use and pregnancy outcome. *Neurobehav Toxicol Teratol* 3:173–181, 1981.

Kaminski, M, Rumeau-Rouquette, C, Schwartz, D: Consommation d'alcool chez les femmes enceintes et issue de la grossesse (Consumption of alcohol among pregnant women and outcome of the pregnancy). *Rev d'Epidemiol Santé Publique* 24:27–40, 1976.

Kellogg, C, Tervc, D, Ison, J, Parisi, T, Miller, RK: Prenatal exposure to diazepam alters behavioral development in rats. *Science* 207:205–207, 1980.

Kesäniemi, YA: Metabolism of ethanol and acetaldehyde in intact rats during pregnancy. *Biochem Pharmacol* 23:1157–1162, 1974.

Kesäniemi, YA, Sippel, HW: Placental and foetal metabolism of acetaldehyde in rat I. Contents of ethanol and acetaldehyde in placenta and foetus of the pregnant rat during ethanol oxidation. *Acta Pharmacol Toxicol* 37:43–48, 1975.

Khan, A, Bader, JL, Hoy, GR, Sinks, LF: Hepatoblastoma in child with fetal alcohol syndrome. *Lancet* 1:1403–1404, 1979.

Kimball, AW: Alcohol and pregnancy (Letter). *Science* 221:1246, 1983.

Kinney, H, Faix, R, Brazy, J: The fetal alcohol syndrome and neuroblastoma. *Pediatrics* 66:130–132, 1980.

Kirkpatrick, SE, Pitlick, PT, Hirschklau, MJ, Friedman, WF: Acute effects of maternal ethanol infusion on fetal cardiac performance. *Am J Obstet Gynecol* 126:1034–1037, 1976.

Kissin, B: Interactions of ethyl alcohol and other drugs. In B Kissin and H Begleiter, eds, *The Biology of Alcoholism, Vol 3, Clinical Pathology*. Plenum Press, New York, 1974, pp. 109–161.

Klassen, RW, Persaud, TVN: Experimental studies on the influence of male alcoholism on pregnancy and progeny. *Exp Pathol* 12:38–45, 1976.

Kline, H, Shrout, P, Stein, Z, Susser, M, Warburton, D: Drinking during pregnancy and spontaneous abortion. *Lancet* 2:176–180, 1980.

Knott, DH, Beard, JD: Effects of alcohol ingestion on the cardiovascular system. In EM Pattison and E Kaufman, eds, *Encyclopedic Handbook of Alcoholism*. New York, Gardner Press, 1982.

Koda, LY, Shoemaker, WJ, Shoemaker, CA: Toxic effects of ethanol on the chicken embryo. *Subst Alcohol Actions Misuse* 1:345–350, 1980.

Kohila, T, Eriksson, K, Halkka, O: Goniomitosis in rats subjected to ethanol. *Med Biol* 54:150–151, 1976.

Kolata, GB: Fetal alcohol advisory debated: some researchers question the government's advice that pregnant women not drink at all. *Science* 214:642–645, 1981.

Korányi, G, Csiky, E: Az embryopathia alcoholica gyermekkorban észlelhető tüneteiről (Signs of alcohol embryopathy apparent in childhood). *Orvosi Hetilap* 119:2923–2929, 1978.

Kornguth, SE, Rutledge, JJ, Sunderland, E, Siegel, F, Carlson, I, Smollens J, Juhl, U, Young, B: Impeded cerebellar development and reduced serum thyroxine levels associated with fetal alcohol intoxication. *Brain Res* 177:347–360, 1979.

Korsten, MA, Matsuzaki, S, Feinman, L, Leiber, CS: High blood acetaldehyde levels after ethanol administration. *N Engl J Med* 292: 386–389, 1975.

Kronick, JB: Teratogenic effects of ethyl alcohol administered to pregnant mice. *Am J Obstet Gynecol* 124:676–680, 1976.

Kurpa, K, Holmberg, PC, Kuosma, E, Saxén, L: Coffee consumption during pregnancy (Letter). *N Eng J Med* 306:1548, 1982.

Kuzma, JW, Kissinger, DG: Patterns of alcohol and cigarette use in pregnancy. *Neurobehav Toxicol Teratol* 3:211–221, 1981.

Kuzma, JW, Sokol, RJ: Maternal drinking behavior and decreased intrauterine growth. *Alcoholism Clin Exp Res* 6:396–402, 1982.

Kyllerman, M, Aronsson, A, Karlberg, E, Olegård, R, Sabel, K-G, Sandin, B, Johansson, PR, Carlsson, C, Iversen, K: Epidemiologic and neuropediatric aspects of the fetal alcohol syndrome. *Neuropadiatrie* 10 (*Suppl*):435–436, 1979.

Landesman-Dwyer, S, Emanuel, I: Smoking during pregnancy. *Teratology* 19:119–126, 1979.

Landesman-Dwyer, S, Keller, LS, Streissguth, AP: Naturalistic observations of newborns: effects of maternal alcohol intake. *Alcoholism Clin Exp Res* 2:171–177, 1978.

Landesman-Dwyer, S, Ragozin, AS, Little, RE: Behavioral correlates of prenatal alcohol exposure: a four-year follow-up study. *Neurobehav Toxicol Teratol* 3:187–194, 1981.

Langman, J: *Medical Embryology: Human Development—Normal and Abnormal*, 3rd ed, Williams and Wilkins, Baltimore, 1975.

Larsson, G: Prevention of fetal alcohol effects: an antenatal program for early detection of pregnancies at risk. *Acta Obstet Gynecol Scand* 62:171–178, 1983.

Lau, C, Thadani, PV, Schanberg, SM, Slotkin, TA: Effects of maternal ethanol ingestion on development of adrenal catecholamines and dopamine-beta-hydroxylase in the offspring. *Neuropharmacology* 15:505–507, 1976.

Leak, AM: Alcohol and the fetus (Letter). *Lancet* 1:984, 1983.

Lefkowitch, JH, Rushton, AR, Feng-Chen, K-C: Hepatic fibrosis in fetal alcohol syndrome: pathologic similarities to adult alcoholic liver disease. *Gastroenterology* 85:951–957, 1983.

Lemoine, P, Harousseau, H, Borteyru, J-P, Menuet, J-C: Les enfants de parents alcooliques: anomalies observées. A propos de 127 cas (Children of alcoholic parents: anomalies observed in 127 cases). *Ouest Med* 21:476–482, 1968.

Lester, D: Endogenous alcohol: a review. *Quart J Stud Alcohol* 22:554–574, 1961.

Lester, D: The concentration of apparent endogenous ethanol. *Quart J Stud Alcohol* 23:17–25, 1962.

Lewis, PJ, Boylan, P: Alcohol and fetal breathing. *Lancet* 1:388, 1979.

Lieber, CS, DeCarli, LM: The role of the hepatic microsomal ethanol oxidizing system (MEOS) for ethanol oxidation in vivo. *J Pharmacol Exp Ther* 181:279–287, 1972.

Lin, GW-J: Fetal malnutrition: a possible cause of the fetal alcohol syndrome. *Prog Biochem Pharmacol* 18:115–121, 1981.

Lindenbaum, J: Hematologic effects of alcohol. In B Kissin, H Begleiter, eds, *The Biology of Alcohol, Vol 3, Clinical Pathology*, Plenum, New York, 1974, pp. 461–480.

Lindenschmidt, RR, Persaud, TVN: Effect of ethanol and nicotine in the pregnant rat. *Res Comm Chem Pathol Pharmacol* 27:195–198, 1980.

Lindros, KO: Regulatory factors in hepatic acetaldehyde metabolism during ethanol oxidation. In KO Lindros and CJP Eriksson, eds, *The Role of Acetaldehyde in the Actions of Ethanol*, Vol 23. Finnish Foundation for Alcohol Studies, 1975, pp. 67–81.

Lindros, KO: Human blood acetaldehyde levels: with improved methods, a clearer picture emerges. *Alcoholism Clin Exp Res* 6:70–75, 1983.

Linn, S, Schoenbaum, S, Monson, RR, Rosner, B, Stubblefield, PG, Ryan, KJ: No association between coffee consumption and adverse outcomes of pregnancy. *N Eng J Med* 306:141–145, 1982.

Lipson, AH, Walsh, DA, Webster, WS: Fetal alcohol syndrome, a great paediatric imitator. *Med J Aust* 1:266–269, 1983.

Little, RE: Moderate alcohol use during pregnancy and decreased infant birth weight. *Am J Public Health* 67:1154–1156, 1977.

Little, RE, Grathwohl, HL, Streissguth, AP, McIntyre, C: Public awareness and knowledge about the risks of drinking during pregnancy in Multnomah County, Oregon. *Am J Pub Health* 71:312–314, 1981.

Little, RE, Mandell, W, Schultz, FA: Consequences of retrospective measurement of alcohol consumption. *J Stud Alcohol* 38:1777–1780, 1977.

Little, RE, Schultz, FA, Mandell, W: Drinking during pregnancy. *J Stud Alcohol* 37:375–379, 1976.

Little, RE, Streissguth, AP: Drinking during pregnancy in alcoholic women. *Alcoholism Clin Exp Res* 2:179–183, 1978.

Little, RE, Streissguth, AP, Barr, HM, Herman, CS: Decreased birth weight in infants of alcoholic women who abstained during pregnancy. *J Pediatr* 96:974–977, 1980a.

Little, RE, Streissguth, AP, Guzinski, GM: Prevention of fetal alcohol syndrome: a model program. *Alcoholism Clin Exp Res* 4:185–189, 1980b.

Little, RE, Streissguth, AP, Guzinski, GM, Grathwohl, HL, Blumhagen, JM, McIntyre, CE: Change in obstetrician advice following a two-year community educational program on alcohol use and pregnancy. *Am J Obstet Gynecol* 146:23–28, 1983.

Little, RE, Streissguth, AP, Page, EL: Techniques for recruiting special types of persons for research: pitfalls and successes in enlisting recovered alcoholic women. *Public Health Reports* 94:332–335, 1979.

Lochry, EA, Randall, CL, Goldsmith, AA, Sutker, PB: Effects of acute alcohol exposure during selected days of gestation in C3H mice. *Neurobehav Toxicol Teratol* 4:15–19, 1982.

Longo, LD: The biologic effects of carbon monoxide on the pregnant woman, fetus, and newborn infant. *Am J Obstet Gynecol* 129:69–103, 1977.

Löser, H, Majewski, F: Type and frequency of cardiac defects in embryo-fetal alcohol syndrome: report of 16 cases. *Br Heart J* 39:1374–1379, 1977.

Lubchenco, LO: *The High Risk Infant,* Saunders, Philadelphia, 1976, pp. 5–12.

MacLusky, NJ, Naftolin, F: Sexual differentiation of the central nervous system. *Science* 211:1294–1302, 1981.

Majewski, F: Die alkoholembryopathie: fakten und hypothesen Ergebninn. *Med Kinderheilk* 43:1–55, 1979.

Majewski, F: Alcohol embryopathy: some facts and speculations about pathogenesis. *Neurobehav Toxicol Teratol* 3:129–144, 1981.

Majewski, F, Fischbach, H, Peiffer, J, Bierich, JR: Zur Frage der Interruptio bei alkoholkranken Frauen (Interruption of pregnancy in alcoholic women). *Deutsche Med Wochenschrift* 103:895–898, 1978.

Mann, LI, Bhakthavanthsalan, A, Liu, M, Makowski, P: Placental transport of alcohol and its effect on maternal and fetal acid-base balance. *Am J Obstet Gynecol* 122:837–844, 1975a.

Mann, LI, Bhakthavathsalan, A, Liu, M, Makowski, P: Effect of alcohol on fetal cerebral function and metabolism. *Am J Obstet Gynecol* 122:845–851, 1975b.

Manzke, H, Grosse, FR: Inkomplettes und komplettes "fetales alkoholsyndrom" bei drei kindern einer trinkerin (Incomplete and complete "fetal alcohol syndrome" in three children of an alcoholic woman). *Die Med Welt* 26:709–712, 1975.

Marbury, MC, Linn, S, Monson, RR, Schoenbaum, SC, Stubblefield, PG, Ryan, KJ: The association of alcohol consumption with outcome of pregnancy. *Am J Public Health* 73:1165–1168, 1983.

Marcus J, Hans, SL: A methodological model to study the effects of toxins on child development. *Neurobehav Toxicol Teratol* 4:483–487, 1982.

Martin, DC, Martin, JC, Streissguth, AP, Lund, CA: Sucking frequency and amplitude in newborns as a function of maternal drinking and smoking. In M Galanter, ed, *Currents in Alcoholism*, Vol V, Grune and Stratton, New York, 1979, pp. 359–366.

Martin, JC, Martin, DC, Lund, CA, Streissguth, AP: Maternal alcohol ingestion and cigarette smoking and their effects on newborn conditioning. *Alcoholism* 1:243–247, 1977.

Martin, JC, Martin, DC, Signan, G, Radow, B: Maternal ethanol consumption and hyperactivity in cross-fostered offspring. *Physiol Psychol* 6:362–365, 1978.

May, PA, Hymbaugh, KJ: A pilot project on fetal alcohol syndrome among American Indians. *Alcohol Health Res World* 7:3–9, 1982/83.

Mayer, J, Black, R, MacDonall, J: Child care in families with an alcohol addicted parent. In FA Seixas, ed, *Currents in Alcoholism*, Vol IV, Grune and Stratton, New York, 1978, pp. 329–338.

Mayfield, D, McLeod, G, Hall, P: The CAGE questionnaire: validation of a new alcoholism screening instrument. *Am J Psychiatry* 131: 1121–1123, 1974.

McClain, CJ, Su, L-C: Zinc deficiency in the alcoholic: a review. *Alcoholism Clin Exp Res* 7:5–10, 1983.

McGivern, RF, Clancy, AN, Mousa, S, Couri, D, Noble, EP: Prenatal alcohol exposure alters enkephalin levels, without affecting ethanol preference. *Life Sci* 34:585–589, 1984.

Meadows, NJ, Ruse, W, Smith, MF, Day, J, Keeling, PWN, Scopes, JW, Thompson, RPH, Bloxam, DL: Zinc and small babies. *Lancet* 2: 1135–1136, 1981.

Mello, NK: Some behavioral and biological aspects of alcohol problems in women. In OJ Kalant, ed, *Alcohol and Drug Problems in Women*, Plenum Press, New York, 1980, pp. 263–298.

Mendelson, J: Biological concomitants of alcoholism (1). *N Eng J Med* 283:24–32, 1970a.

Mendelson, J: Biological concomitants of alcoholism (2). *N Eng J Med* 283:71–81, 1970b.

Merkatz, IR, Peter, JB, Barden, TP: Ritodrine hydrochloride: a betamimetric agent for use in preterm labor II. Evidence of efficacy. *Obstet Gynecol* 56:7–12, 1980.

Miller, HC, Merritt, TA: *Fetal Growth in Humans.* Year Book Medical Publishers, Inc., Chicago, 1979, pp. 25–30.

Miller, M: Letter. *Pediatrics* 70:322, 1982.

Minor, M, Van Dort, B: Prevention research on the teratogenic effects of alcohol. *Preventive Med* 11:346–359, 1982.

Møller, J, Brandt, NJ, Tygstrup, I: Hepatic dysfunction in patient with fetal alcohol syndrome. *Lancet* 1:605–6, 1979.

Monjan, AA, Mandell, W: Fetal alcohol and immunity: depression of mitrogen-induced lymphocyte blastogenesis. *Neurobehav Toxicol* 2:213–216, 1980.

Mukherjee, AB, Hodgen, GD: Maternal ethanol exposure induces transient impairment of umbilical circulation and fetal hypoxia in monkeys. *Science* 218:700–702, 1982.

Mulvihill, JJ: Caffeine as teratogen and mutagen. *Teratology* 8:68–72, 1973.

Murphy, HB: Hidden barriers to the diagnosis and treatment of alcoholism and other alcohol misuse. *J Stud Alcohol* 41:417–428, 1980.

Nanson, J, Habbick, BF, Casey, RE, Zaleski, WA: Fetal alcohol syndrome in Saskatchewan: some preliminary findings. *Perinatal Bull* 14: 3–4, 1981.

National Foundation, March of Dimes, *Birth Defects, Abstracts of Selected Articles* 5:11, 1968.

Nelson, LR, Lewis, JW, Liebeskind, JC, Branch, BJ, Taylor, AN: Stress induced changes in ethanol consumption in adult rats exposed to ethanol in utero. *Proc West Pharmacol Soc* 26:205–209, 1983.

Neugut, RH: Epidemiological appraisal of the literature on the fetal alcohol syndrome in humans. *Early Human Dev* 5:411–429, 1981.

Neugut, RH: Fetal alcohol syndrome: how good is the evidence? *Neurobehav Toxicol Teratol* 4:593–594, 1982.

Newman, SL, Flannery, DB, Caplan, DB: Simultaneous occurrence of extrahepatic biliary atresia and fetal alcohol syndrome. *Am J Dis Child* 133:101, 1979.

Nichols, MM: Acute alcohol withdrawal syndrome in a newborn. *Am J Dis Child* 113:714–715, 1967.

Nicloux, M: Passage de l'alcool ingéré de la mère au foetus et passage de l'alcool ingéré dans le lait, en particulier chez la femme. ((Passage of alcohol ingested by the mother to the fetus and passage of alcohol ingested in milk, particularly in women.) *Obstetrique* 5:97–132, 1900.

Nomura, F, Lieber, CS: Binding of acetaldehyde to rat liver microsomes: enhancement after chronic alcohol consumption. *Biochem Biophys Res Commun* 100:131–137, 1981.

Noonan, JA: Congenital heart disease in the fetal alcohol syndrome. *Am J Cardiol* 37:160, 1976.

Nora, AH, Nora, JI, Blu, J: Limb-reduction anomalies in infants born to disulfiram-treated alcoholic mothers. *Lancet* 2:664, 1977.

Øisund, JF, Fjorden, A-E, Morland, J: Is moderate ethanol consumption teratogenic in the rat? *Acta Pharmacol Toxicol* 43:145–155, 1978.

Olegård, R, Johansson, PR, Kyllerman, M, Sabel, K-G: Alkohol och graviditet. *Lakartidningen* 74:37, 1977.

Olegård, R, Sabel, K-G, Aronsson, M, Sandin, B, Johansson, PR, Carlsson, C, Kyllerman, M, Iversen, K, Hrbek, A: Effects on the child of alcohol abuse during pregnancy: retrospective and prospective studies. *Acta Paediatr Scand (Suppl)* 275:112–121, 1979.

Opinion Research Corporation. Public perceptions of alcohol consumption and pregnancy. A nationwide survey conducted for the Bureau of Alcohol, Tobacco, and Firearms. ORC Study No 33710, Princeton, New Jersey, 1979.

Osborne, GL, Caul, WF, Fernandez, K: Behavioral effects of prenatal ethanol exposure and differential early experience in rats. *Pharmacol Biochem Behav* 12:393–401, 1980.

O'Shea, KS, Kaufman, MH: Effect of acetaldehyde on the neuroepithelium of early mouse embryos. *J Anat* 132:107–118, 1981.

O'Shea, KS, Kaufman, MH: The teratogenic effect of acetaldehyde: implications for the study of the fetal alcohol syndrome. *J Anat* 128:65–76, 1979.

Ottinger, D, Simmons, J: Behavior of human neonates and prenatal maternal anxiety. *Psychol Rep* 14:391–394, 1964.

Ouellette, EM, Rosett, HL, Rosman, NP, Weiner, L: The adverse effects on offspring of maternal alcohol abuse during pregnancy. *N Engl J Med* 297:528–530, 1977.

Page, EW, Villee, CA, Villee, DB: *Human Reproduction: The Core Content of Obstetrics, Gynecology, and Perinatal Medicine,* 2d ed, WB Saunders Co, Philadelphia, 1976.

Palmer, HP, Ouellette, EM, Warner, L, Leichtman, SR: Congenital malformations in offspring of a chronic alcoholic mother. *Pediatrics* 53:490–494, 1974.

Parke, RD: Perspectives on father–infant interaction. In JD Osofsky, ed, *Handbook of Infant Development.* John Wiley & Sons, New York, 1979, pp. 549–590.

Peiffer, J, Majewski, F, Fischbach, H, Bierich, JR, Volk, B: Alcohol embryo- and fetopathy: neuropathology of 3 children and 3 fetuses. *J Neurol Sci* 41:125–137, 1979.

Pennington, SN, Smith, CP, Tapscott, EB: Effect of an acute dose of ethanol on rat liver microsomal mixed function oxygenase components and membrane lipid composition. *Alcoholism Clin Exp Res* 2:311–316, 1978.

Persaud, TVN: Further studies on the interaction of ethanol and nicotine in the pregnant rat. *Res Commun Chem Pathol Pharmacol* 37:313–316, 1982.

Persaud, TVN: Prenatal loss in the rat following moderate consumption of alcohol incorporated in a liquid diet. *Anat Anz Jena* 153:169–174, 1983.

Petersen, DR, Panter, SS, Collins, AC: Ethanol and acetaldehyde metabolism in the pregnant mouse. *Drug Alcohol Depend* 2:409–420, 1977.

Phillips, SC, Cragg, BG: A change in susceptibility of rat cerebellar purkinje cells to damage by alcohol during fetal, neonatal and adult life. *Neuropathol Appl Neurobiol* 8:441–454, 1982.

Phillips, M, McAloon, MH: A sweat-patch test for alcohol consumption: evaluation in continuous and episodic drinkers. *Alcoholism Clin Exp Res* 4:391–395, 1980.

Pierog, S, Chandavasu, O, Wexler, I: Withdrawal symptoms in infants with the fetal alcohol syndrome. *J Pediatr* 90:630–633, 1977.

Pittman, DJ: Primary prevention of alcohol abuse: five models of social control. In *Primary Prevention of Alcohol Abuse and Alcoholism*, Social Science Institute, Washington University, St. Louis, 1980, pp. 11–16.

Podratz, KC: Alcohol ketoacidosis in pregnancy. *Obstet Gynecol* 52:54s–57s, 1978.

Polacsek, E, Barnes, T, Turner, N, Hall, R, Weise, C: Interaction of Alcohol and Other Drugs. Addiction Research Foundation, Toronto, Canada, 1972.

Polich, JM: The validity of self-reports in alcoholism research. *Addictive Behav* 7:123–132, 1982.

Ponte, C, Weill, J, Dubos, JP, Gosselin, B, Farine, MO: Sympathoblastome et foetopathie alcoolique: présentation d'une observation. *Med et Hyg* 40:613–616, 1982.

Popov, VB, Vaisman, BL, Puchkov, VF, Ignatyeva, TV: Embryotoxic effect of ethanol and biotransformation products in the culture of postimplantation rat embryos. *Biull Eksp Biol Med* 92:725–728, 1981.

Poskitt, EME, Hensey, OJ, Smith, CS: Alcohol, other drugs and the fetus. *Dev Med Child Neurol* 24:596–602, 1982.

Potter, BJ, Belling, GB, Mano, MT, Hetzel, BS: Experimental production of growth retardation in the sheep fetus after exposure to alcohol. *Med J Aust* 2:191–193, 1980.

Pratt, OE: The fetal alcohol syndrome: transport of nutrients and transfer of alcohol and acetaldehyde from mother to fetus. In *Psychopharmacology of Alcohol*, M. Sandler, ed, Raven Press, New York, 1980, pp. 229–256.

Püschel, K, Seifert, H: Bedeutung des alkohols in der embryofetalperiode und beim neugeborenen (Effects of alcohol in the embryo, fetus, and newborn infant). *Zeitschrift fur Rechtsmedizin* 83:69–76, 1979.

Qazi, QH, Masakawa, A, McGann, B, Woods, J: Dermatoglyphic abnormalities in the fetal alcohol syndrome. *Teratology* 21:157–160, 1980.

Qazi, Q, Masakawa, A, Milman, D, McGann, B, Chua, A, Haller, J: Renal anomalies in fetal alcohol syndrome. *Pediatrics* 63:886–889, 1979.

Rabinowicz, IM: Opthalmologic findings in the foetal alcohol syndrome. *Opthalmology* 87 (Suppl):93, 1980.

Ragozin, AS, Landesman-Dwyer, S, Streissguth, AP: The relationship between mothers' drinking habits and children's home environments. In M Galanter, ed, *Currents in Alcoholism*, Vol 4. Grune and Stratton, New York, 1978, pp. 39–49.

Rainey, JM: Disulfiram toxicity and carbon disulfide poisoning. *Am J Psychiatry* 134:371–378, 1977.

Ramilo, J, Harris, VJ: Neuroblastoma in a child with the hydantoin and fetal alcohol syndrome. *Br J Radiol* 52:993–995, 1979.

Randall, C: Alcohol as a teratogen in animals. In *Biomedical Processes and Consequences of Alcohol Use*, Alcohol and Health Monograph 2, DHHS, 1982, pp. 291–307.

Randall, CL, Burling, TA, Lochry, EA, Sutker, PB: The effect of paternal alcohol consumption on fetal development in mice. *Drug Alcohol Depend* 9:89–95, 1982.

Randall, CL, Lochry EA, Hughes, SS, Sutker, PB: Dose-response effect of prenatal alcohol exposure on fetal growth and development in mice. *Substance and Alcohol Actions/Misuse* 2:349–357, 1981.

Randall, CL, Riley, EP: Prenatal alcohol exposure: current issues and the status of animal research. *Neurobehav Toxicol Teratol* 3:111–115, 1981.

Randall, CL, Taylor, WJ: Prenatal ethanol exposure in mice: teratogenic effects. *Teratology* 19:305–312, 1979.

Randall, CL, Taylor, WJ, Tabakoff, B, Walker, BW: Ethanol as a teratogen. In RB Thurman, JR Williamson, HR Drott, B Chance, eds, *Alcohol and Aldehyde Metabolizing Systems, Vol III, Intermediary Metabolism and Neurochemistry*. Academic Press, New York, 1977a, pp. 659–670.

Randall, CL, Taylor, WJ, Walker, DW: Ethanol-induced malformations in mice. *Alcoholism Clin Exp Res* 1:219–224, 1977b.

Rasmussen, BR, Christensen, N: Teratogenic effect of maternal alcohol consumption on the mouse fetus. *Acta Path Microbiol Scand 88A:* 285–289, 1980.

Rawat, AK: Developmental changes in the brain levels of neurotransmitters as influenced by maternal ethanol consumption in the rat. *J Neurochem 28:*1175–1182, 1977.

Rawat, AK: Derangement in cardiac protein metabolism in fetal alcohol syndrome. *Res Commun Chem Pathol Pharmacol 25:*365–375, 1979.

Rawat, AK: Psychotropic drug metabolism in fetal alcohol syndrome. *Adv Exp Med Biol 132:*561–568, 1980.

Revill, SI, Dodge, JA: Psychological determinants of infantile pyloric stenosis. *Arch Dis Child 53:*66–68, 1978.

Riley, EP: Ethanol as a behavioral teratogen: animal models. In *Biomedical Processes and Consequences of Alcohol Use,* Alcohol and Health Monograph 2, DHHS, 1982, pp. 311–332.

Riley, EP, Lochry, EA: Genetic influences in the etiology of fetal alcohol syndrome. In EL Abel, ed, *Fetal Alcohol Syndrome* Vol III, CRC Press, Boca Raton, Florida, 1982, pp. 113–130.

Riley, EP, Lochry, EA, Shapiro, NR: Lack of response inhibition in rats prenatally exposed to alcohol. *Psychopharmocology 62:*47–52, 1979a.

Riley, EP, Lochry, EA, Shapiro, NR, Baldwin, J: Response perseveration in rats exposed to alcohol prenatally. *Pharmacol Biochem Behav 10:*255–259, 1979b.

Riley, EP, Shapiro, NR, Lochry, EA: Nose-poking and head-dipping behaviors in rats prenatally exposed to alcohol. *Pharmacol Biochem Behav 11:*513–519, 1979c.

Robe, LB, Robe, RS, Wilson, A: Maternal heavy drinking related to delayed onset of daughters' menstruation. *Alcoholism Clin Exp Res 3:*192, 1979.

Root, AW, Reiter, EO, Andriola, M, Duckett, G: Hypothalamic-pituitary function in the fetal alcohol syndrome. *J Pediatr 87:*585–587, 1975.

Rose, JC, Meis, PJ, Castro, MI: Alcohol and fetal endocrine function. *Neurobehav Toxicol Teratol 3:*105–110, 1981.

Rosett, HL: Maternal alcoholism and intellectual development of offspring (Letter). *Lancet 2:*218, 1974.

Rosett, HL: A clinical perspective of the fetal alcohol syndrome. *Alcoholism Clin Exp Res 4:*119–122, 1980a.

Rosett, HL: The effects of alcohol on the fetus and offspring. In OJ Kalant, ed, *Alcohol and Drug Problems in Women,* Plenum, New York, 1980b, pp. 595–652.

Rosett, HL, Ouellette, EM, Weiner, L, Owens, E: Therapy of heavy drinking during pregnancy. *Obstet Gynecol* 51:41–46, 1978.

Rosett, HL, Snyder, PA, Sander, LW, Lee, A, Cook, P, Weiner, L, Gould, J: Effects of maternal drinking on neonate state regulation. *Dev Med Child Neurol* 21:464–473, 1979.

Rosett, HL, Weiner, L: Clinical and experimental perspectives on prevention of the fetal alcohol syndrome. *Neurobehav Toxicol* 2:267–270, 1980.

Rosett, HL, Weiner, L: Identifying and treating pregnant patients at risk from alcohol. *Can Med Assoc J* 125:149–154, 1981.

Rosett, HL, Weiner, L: Commentary: prevention of fetal alcohol effects. *Pediatrics* 69:813–816, 1982.

Rosett, HL, Weiner, L, Edelin, KC: Strategies for prevention of fetal alcohol effects. *Obstet Gynecol* 57:1–7, 1981.

Rosett, HL, Weiner, L, Edelin, KC: Treatment experience with pregnant problem drinkers. *J Am Med Assoc* 249:2029–2033, 1983a.

Rosett, HL, Weiner, L, Lee, A, Zuckerman, B, Dooling, E, Oppenheimer, E: Patterns of alcohol consumption and fetal development. *Obstet Gynecol* 61:539–546, 1983b.

Rosett, HL, Weiner, L, Zuckerman, B, McKinlay, S, Edelin, KC: Reduction of alcohol consumption during pregnancy with benefits to the newborn. *Alcoholism Clin Exp Res* 4:178–184, 1980.

Russell, M: Screening for alcohol related problems in obstetric and gynecologic patients. In EL Abel, ed, *Fetal Alcohol Syndrome*, Vol II, CRC Press, Boca Raton, Florida, 1982a, pp. 1–19.

Ruth, RE, Goldsmith, SK: Interaction between zinc deprivation and acute ethanol intoxication during pregnancy in rats. *J Nutr* 111:2034–2038, 1981.

Sameroff, AJ, Chandler, MJ: Reproductive risk and the continuum of caretaking casuality. In FD Horowitz, ed, *Review of Child Development Research*, Vol 4, University of Chicago Press, Chicago, 1975, pp. 187–243.

Samson, HH, Grant, KA: Ethanol induced microcephaly in the neonatal rat: relation to dose. *Alcoholism Clin Exp Res* 7:120, 1983.

Samson, HH, Waterman, DL, Woods, SC: Effect of acute maternal ethanol exposure upon fetal development in the rat. *Physiol Psychol* 7:311–315, 1979.

Sander, LW, Snyder, PA, Rosett, HL, Lee, A, Gould, JB, Ouellette, EM: Effects of alcohol intake during pregnancy on newborn state regulation: a progress report. *Alcoholism Clin Exp Res* 1:233–241, 1977.

Sandor, GGS, Smith, DF, MacLeod, PM: Cardiac malformations in the fetal alcohol syndrome. *J Pediatr* 98:771–773, 1981.

Sandor, S, Checiu, M, Fazakas-Todea, I, Garbân, Z: The effect of ethanol upon early development in mice and rats. I. In vivo effect upon preimplantation and early postimplantation stages. *Morphol Embryol* 26:265–274, 1980.

Santolaya, JM, Martinez, G, Gorostiza, E, Aizpiri, J, Hernandez, M: Alcoholismo fetal (Fetal alcohol syndrome). *Drogalchol* 3:183–192, 1978.

Schaefer, O: Alcohol withdrawal syndrome in a newborn infant of a Yukon Indian mother. *Can Med Assoc J* 87:1333–1334, 1962.

Scheiner, AP: Fetal alcohol syndrome in a child whose parents had stopped drinking. *Lancet* 2:858, 1979.

Scheiner, AP, Donovan, CM, Bartoshesky, LE: Fetal alcohol syndrome in child whose parents had stopped drinking. *Lancet* 1:1077–1078, 1979.

Schwetz, BA, Smith, FA, Staples, RE: Teratogenic potential of ethanol in mice, rats, and rabbits. *Teratology* 18:385–392, 1978.

Scott, WJ: Cell death and reduced proliferative rate. In JG Wilson and FC Fraser, eds, *Handbook of Teratology*, Vol II, Plenum Press, New York, 1977, pp. 81–98.

Seeler, RA, Israel, JN, Royal, JE, Kaye, CI, Rao, S, Abulaban, M: Ganglioneuroblastoma and fetal hydantoin-alcohol syndromes. *Pediatrics* 63:524–527, 1979.

Seidenberg, J, Majewski, F: Zur Haeufigkeit der Alkoholembryopathie in den Verschiedenen Phasen der muetterlichen Alkoholkrankheit. (Frequency of alcohol embryopathy in the different phases of maternal alcoholism). *Hamburg Suchtgefahren* 24:63–75, 1978.

Sellers, EM, Busto, U: Benzodiazepines and ethanol: assessment of the effects and consequences of psychotropic drug interactions. *J Clin Psychopharmacol* 2:249–262, 1982.

Selzer, ML: The Michigan Alcoholism Screening Test: the quest for a new diagnostic instrument. *Am J Psychiatry* 127:1653–1658, 1971.

Seppälä, M, Fäihä, NCR, Tamminen, V: Ethanol elimination in a mother and her premature twins. *Lancet* 1:1188–1189, 1971.

Shaywitz, SE, Caparulo, BK, Hodgson, ES: Developmental language disability as a consequence of prenatal exposure to ethanol. *Pediatrics* 68:850–855, 1981.

Shaywitz, SE, Caparulo, BK, Hodgson, ES: Letter. *Pediatrics* 70:324–325, 1982.

Shaywitz, SE, Cohen, DJ, Shaywitz, BA: Behavior and learning difficulties in children of normal intelligence born to alcoholic mothers. *J Pediatr* 96:978–982, 1980.

Shaywitz, BA, Klopper, JH, Gordon, JW: A syndrome resembling minimal brain dysfunction (MBD) in rat pups born to alcoholic mothers. *Pediatr Res 10*:451, 1976.

Sheean, LA: Aromatization of androstenedione by microsomes from the human placenta after gestational alcohol consumption. *Alcoholism Clin Exp Res 7*:93–94, 1983.

Shibutani, K: Anesthetic management of the alcoholic patient. In AB Lowenfels, ed, *The Alcoholic Patient in Surgery,* Williams and Wilkins, Baltimore, 1971, pp. 67–79.

Shoemaker, WJ, Baetge, G, Azad, R, Sapin, V, Bloom, FE: Effect of prenatal alcohol exposure on amine and peptide neurotransmitter systems. *Monogr Neural Sci 9*:130–139, 1983.

Shurygin, GI: Ob osobennostyakh psikhicheskogo razvitiya detey ot materey, stradayushchikh khronicheskim alkogolizmom (Characteristics of the mental development of children of chronic alcoholic mothers). *Pediatriya 11*:71–73, 1974.

Silva, VA, Laranjeira, RR, Dolnikoff, M, Grinfeld, H, Masur, J: Alcohol consumption during pregnancy and newborn outcome: a study in Brazil. *Neurobehav Toxicol Teratol 3*:169–172, 1981.

Skosyreva, AM: Vliyaniye etilovogo spirta na razvitiye embrionov stadii organogeneza (Effect of ethyl alcohol on embryo development at the stage of organogenesis). *Akush Ginekol (Moskow) 4*:15–18, 1973.

Smith, DF, MacLeod, PM, Tredwell, S, Wood, B, Newman, DE: Intrinsic defects in the fetal alcohol syndrome: studies on 76 cases from British Columbia and the Yukon Territory. *Neurobehav Toxicol Teratol 3*:145–152, 1981.

Smith, DW, Gong, BT: Scalp-hair patterning: its origins and significance relative to early brain and upper facial development. *Teratology 9*:17–34, 1974.

Smith, DW, Graham, JM: Fetal alcohol syndrome in a child whose parents had stopped drinking (Letter). *Lancet 2*:527, 1979.

Snow, MHL, Tam, PPL: Is compensatory growth a complicating factor in mouse teratology? *Nature 279*:555–557, 1979.

Sokol, RJ: Alcohol and spontaneous abortion (Letter). *Lancet 2*:1079, 1980.

Sokol, RJ: Alcohol and abnormal outcomes of pregnancy. *Can Med Assoc J 125*:143–148, 1981.

Sokol, RJ, Gross, T, Chik, LC, Halvorsen, P, Williams, T: Maternal drinking and fetal lung maturation. *Proc Ann Meet Soc Perinatal Obstet,* January 1983, San Antonio, p. 35A.

Sokol, RJ, Miller, SI: Identifying the alcohol abusing obstetric/gynecologic patient: a practical approach. *Alcohol Health Res World 4*:36–40, 1980.

Sokol, RJ, Miller, SI, Debanne, S, Golden, N, Collins, G, Kaplan, J, Martier, S: The Cleveland NIAAA prospective alcohol-in-pregnancy study: the first year. *Neurobehav Toxicol Teratol* 3:203–209, 1981.

Sokol, RJ, Miller, SI, Reed, G: Alcohol abuse during pregnancy: an epidemiological model. *Alcoholism Clin Exp Res* 4:135–145, 1980.

Sonderegger, TB, Calmes, H, Corbitt, S, and Zimmerman, EG: Lack of persistent effect of low-dose ethanol administered postnatally in rats. *Neurobehav Toxicol Teratol* 4:463–468, 1982.

Spiegel, PG, Pekman, WM, Rich, BH, Versteeg, CN, Nelson, V, Dudnikov, M: The orthopedic aspects of the fetal alcohol syndrome. *Clin Orthop* 139:58–63, 1979.

Sprung, R, Bonte, W, Rüdell, E, Domke, M, Frauenrath, C: Sum Problem des endogenen Alkohols (Endogenous ethanol: further investigations). *Blutalkohol* 18:65–70, 1981.

Sreenathan, RN, Padmanabhan, R, Singh, S: Teratogenic effects of acetaldehyde in the rat. *Drug Alcohol Depend* 9:339–350, 1982.

Stechler, G, Halton, A: Prenatal influences on human development. In B Wolman, ed, *Handbook of Developmental Psychology*, Prentice-Hall, 1982, pp. 175–189.

Steeg, CN, Woolf, P: Cardiovascular malformations in the fetal alcohol syndrome. *Am Heart J* 98:635–637, 1979.

Stein, Z, Kline, J: Smoking, alcohol and reproduction (Editorial). *Am J Public Health* 73:1154–1156, 1983.

Steinhausen, H-C, Nestler, V, Spohr, H-L: Development and psychopathology of children with the fetal alcohol syndrome. *Dev Behav Ped* 3:49–54, 1982.

Stott, DH, Latchford, SA: Prenatal antecedents of child health, development, and behavior: an epidemiological report of incidence and association. *J Am Acad Child Psychiat* 15:161–191, 1976.

Streissguth, AP, Barr, HM, Martin, DC: Maternal alcohol use and neonatal habituation assessed with the Brazelton Scale. *Child Dev* 54:1109–1118, 1983a.

Streissguth, AP, Barr, HM, Martin, DC: Offspring effects and pregnancy complications related to self-reported maternal alcohol use. *Dev Pharmacol Ther* 5:21–32, 1982.

Streissguth, AP, Barr, HM, Martin, DC, Herman, CS: Effects of maternal alcohol, nicotine, and caffeine use during pregnancy on infant mental and motor development at eight months. *Alcoholism Clin Exp Res* 4:152–164, 1980.

Streissguth, AP, Darby, BL, Barr, HM, Smith, JR, Martin, DC: Comparison of drinking and smoking patterns during pregnancy over a six-year interval. *Am J Obstet Gynecol* 145:716–724, 1983b.

Streissguth, AP, Herman, CS, Smith, DW: Intelligence, behavior, and dysmorphogenesis in the fetal alcohol syndrome: a report on 20 patients. *J Pediatr* 92:363–367, 1978a.

Streissguth, AP, Herman, CS, Smith, DW: Stability of intelligence in the fetal alcohol syndrome: a preliminary report. *Alcoholism Clin Exp Res* 2:165–170, 1978b.

Streissguth, AP, Martin, DC, Martin, JC, and Barr, HM: The Seattle longitudinal prospective study on alcohol and pregnancy. *Neurobehav Toxicol Teratol* 3:223–233, 1981.

Strömland, K: Eyeground malformations in the fetal alcohol syndrome. *Neuropediatrics* 12:97–98, 1981.

Sudman, S, Bradburn, NM: Response effects in surveys: a review and synthesis. NORC Monographs in Social Research Series No. 16, 1974.

Sulik, KK, Johnston, MC: Embryonic origin of holoprosencephaly: interrelationship of the developing brain and face. *Scanning Electron Microsc* 1:309–322, 1982.

Sulik, KK, Johnston, MC: Sequence of developmental alterations following acute ethanol exposure in mice: craniofacial features of the fetal alcohol syndrome. *Am J Anat* 166:257–269, 1983.

Sulik, KK, Johnston, MC, Webb, MA: Fetal alcohol syndrome: embryogenesis in a mouse model. *Science* 214:936–938, 1981.

Sullivan, LW: Folates in human nutrition. In AA Albanese, ed, *Newer Methods of Nutritional Biochemistry*, Vol III, Academic Press, New York, 1967, pp. 365–406.

Sullivan, LW, Herbert, V: Suppression of hematopoiesis by ethanol. *J Clin Invest* 43:2048–2062, 1964.

Sullivan, WC: A note on the influence of maternal inebriety on the offspring. *J Ment Sci* 45:489–503, 1899.

Surgeon General's advisory on alcohol and pregnancy. *FDA Drug Bull* 11:9–10, 1981.

Tanaka, H, Arima, M, Suzuki, N: The fetal alcohol syndrome in Japan. *Brain Dev* 3:305–311, 1981.

Tanaka, H, Nakazawa, K, Suzuki, N, Arima, M: Prevention possibility for brain dysfunction in rat with the fetal alcohol syndrome: low-zinc-status and hypoglycemia. *Brain Dev* 4:429–438, 1982.

Tanaka, H, Suzuki, N, Arima, M: Experimental studies on the influence of male alcoholism on fetal development. *Brain Dev* 4:1–6, 1982a.

Tanaka, H, Suzuki, N, Arima, M: Hypoglycemia in the fetal alcohol syndrome in rat. *Brain Dev* 4:97–103, 1982b.

Taylor, AN, Branch, BJ, Kokka, N: Neuroendocrine effects of fetal alcohol exposure. *Prog Biochem Pharmacol* 18:99–110, 1981.

Taylor, AN, Branch, BJ, Kokka, N, Poland, RE: Neonatal and long-term neuroendocrine effects of fetal alcohol exposure. *Mongr Neural Sci* 9:140–152, 1983.

Tenbrinck, MS, Buchin, SY: Fetal alcohol syndrome: a report of a case. *J Am Med Assoc* 232:1144–1147, 1975.

Tennes, K, Blackard, C: Maternal alcohol consumption, birth weight, and minor physical anomalies. *Am J Obstet Gynecol* 138:774–780, 1980.

Thadani, PV, Schanberg, SM: Effect of maternal ethanol ingestion on serum growth hormone in the developing rat. *Neuropharmacology* 18:821–826, 1979.

Thadani, PV, Slotkin, TA, Schanberg, SM: Effects of late prenatal or early postnatal ethanol exposure on ornithine decarboxylase activity in brain and heart of developing rats. *Neuropharmacology* 16:289–293, 1977.

Tissot-Favre, M, Delatour, P: Psychopharmacologie et teratogenese à propos du disulfirame: essai experimental (Psychopharmacology and teratogenicity of disulfiram: an experimental study). *Ann Med Psychol* 1:735–740, 1965.

Tittmar, H-G: Some effects of ethanol, presented during the prenatal period on the development of rats. *Br J Alcohol Alcoholism* 12: 71–83, 1977.

Toutant, C, Lippman, S: Fetal solvents syndrome (Letter). *Lancet 1*: 1356, 1979.

Tredwell, SJ, Smith, DF, Macleod, PJ, Wood, BJ: Cervical spine anomalies in fetal alcohol syndrome. *Spine* 7:331–334, 1982.

Tremblay, PC, Sybulski, S, Maughan, GB: Role of the placenta in fetal malnutrition. *Am J Obstet Gynecol* 91:597–605, 1965.

Truitt, EB, Walsh, MJ: The role of acetaldehyde in the actions of ethanol. In B Kissen and H Begleiter, eds, *The Biology of Alcohol, Vol I, Biochemistry*. Plenum, New York 1971, pp. 161–195.

Tze, WJ, Friesen, HG, MacLeod, PM: Growth hormone response in fetal alcohol syndrome. *Arch Dis Child* 51:703–706, 1976.

U.S. Department of Health and Human Services: Alcohol and Health. Fourth Special Report to the U.S. Congress, U.S. Government Printing Office, Washington, D.C., 1981.

U.S. Department of Health, Education and Welfare: Alcohol and Health. Third Special Report to the U.S. Congress, U.S. Government Printing Office, Washington D.C., 1978.

U.S. Department of the Treasury, Bureau of Alcohol, Tobacco and Firearms. Report to the President and the Congress on health hazards associated with alcohol and methods to inform the general public of these hazards. U.S. Government Printing Office, Washington, D.C., 1980.

Ulleland, C, Wennberg, RP, Igo, RP, Smith, NJ: The offspring of alcoholic mothers. *Pediatr Res* 4:474, 1970.

Valente, M: Letter. *Pediatrics* 70:323, 1982.

Van Dyke, DC, Mackay, L, Ziaylek, EN: Management of severe feeding dysfunction in children with fetal alcohol syndrome. *Clin Pediatr* 21:336–339, 1982.

Van Thiel, DH, Gavaler, JS: The adverse effects of ethanol upon hypothalamic-pituitary-gonadal function in males and females compared and contrasted. *Alcoholism Clin Exp Res* 6:179–185, 1982.

Van Thiel, DH, Gavaler, JS, Lester, R: Ethanol: a gonadal toxin in the female. *Drug Alcohol Depend* 2:373–380, 1977.

Varma, PK, Persaud, TVN: Influence on pyrazole, an inhibitor of alcohol dehydrogenase, on the prenatal toxicity of ethanol in the rat. *Res Commun Chem Pathol Pharmacol* 26:65–73, 1979.

Varma, PK, Persaud, TVN: Protection against ethanol-induced embryonic damage by administering gamma linolenic and linoleic acids. *Prostaglandins Leukotrienes Med* 8:641–645, 1982.

Véghelyi, PV, Osztovics, M: Fetal-alcohol syndrome in child whose parents had stopped drinking (Letter). *Lancet* 2:35–36, 1979.

Véghelyi, PV, Osztovics, M, Kardos, G, Leisztner, L, Szaszovszky, E, Igali, S, Imrei, J: The fetal alcohol syndrome: symptoms and pathogenesis. *Acta Paediatr Acad Sci Hung* 19:171–189, 1978.

Volk, B: Verzögerte kleinhirnentwicklung im rahmen des "embryofetalen alkoholsydroms." *Acta Neuropathol (Berl)* 39:157–163, 1977.

Volk, B, Maletz, J, Tiedemann, M, Mall, G, Klein, C, Berlet, HH: Impaired maturation of Purkinje cells in the fetal alcohol syndrome of the rat: light and electron microscopic investigations. *Acta Neuropathol* 54:19–29, 1981.

von Wartburg, J-P: The metabolism of alcohol in normals and alcoholics: enzymes. In B Kissin and H Begleiter, eds, *The Biology of Alcoholism, Vol I, Biochemistry.* Plenum Press, New York, 1971, pp. 63–102.

von Wartburg, J-P: Acetaldehyde. In M Sandler, ed, *Psychopharmacology of Alcohol.* Raven Press, New York, 1980, pp. 137–147.

Wagman, AMI, Allen, RP: Effects of alcohol ingestion and abstinence on slow wave sleep of alcoholics. *Adv Exp Med Biol* 59:453–466, 1975.

Wagner, G, Fuchs, A-R: Effect of ethanol on uterine activity during suckling in post-partum women. *Acta Endocrinol (Copenhagen)* 58:133–141, 1968.

Wallgren, H, Barry, H: *Actions of Alcohol,* Vol 2. Elsevier, Amsterdam, 1970, pp. 482–489.

Waltman, R, Iniquez, F, Iniquez, ES: Placental transfer of ethanol and its elimination at term. *Obstet Gynecol* 40:180–185, 1972.

Warner, RH, Rosett, HL: The effects of drinking on offspring: an historical survey of the American and British literature. *J Stud Alcohol* 36:1395–1420, 1975.

Webster, WS, Walsh, DA, Lipson, AH, McEwen, SE: Teratogenesis after acute alcohol exposure in inbred and outbred mice. *Neurobehav Toxicol* 2:227–234, 1980.

Webster, WS, Walsh, DA, McEwen, SE, Lipson, AH: Some teratogenic properties of ethanol and acetaldehyde in C57 BL/6J mice: implications for the study of the fetal alcohol syndrome. *Teratology* 27:231–243, 1983.

Weiner, L, Rosett, HL, and Edelin, KC: Behavioral evaluation of fetal alcohol education for physicians. *Alcoholism Clin Exp Res* 6:230–233, 1982.

Weiner, L, Rosett, HL, Edelin, KC, Alpert, JJ, Zuckerman, B: Alcohol consumption by pregnant women. *Obstet Gynecol* 61:6–12, 1983.

West, JR, Hodges, CA, Black, AC: Prenatal exposure to ethanol alters the organization of hippocampal mossy fibers in rats. *Science 211*: 957–959, 1981.

Whiting, M, Whitman, S, Bergner, L, Patrick, S: Addiction and low birthweight: a quasi-experimental study. *Am J Public Health 68*: 676–678, 1978.

Wilker, R, Nathenson, G: Combined fetal alcohol and hydantoin syndromes. *Clin Pediatr* 21:331–334, 1982.

Wilson, JG: *Environment and Birth Defects.* Academic Press, New York, 1973.

Wilson, KH, Landesman, R, Fuchs, A-R, Fuchs, F: The effect of ethyl alcohol on isolated human myometrium. *Am J Obstet Gynecol* 104:436–439, 1969.

Woodson, PM, Ritchey, SJ: Effect of maternal alcohol consumption on fetal brain cell number and cell size. *Nutrition Rept Int* 20:225–228, 1979.

Wright, JT, Barrison, IG, Lewis, IG, MacRae, KD, Waterson, EJ, Toplis, PJ, Gordon, MG, Morris, NF, Murray-Lyon, IM: Alcohol consumption, pregnancy, and low birthweight. *Lancet* 1:663–665, 1983.

Wuthrich, P, Hauserr, H: *Der Schweitzerische Alkoholkonsum* (Alcohol Consumption in Switzerland). Arbeitsberichte der Forschungsabteilung SFA, Lausanne, 1977.

Yanai, J, Ginsburg, BE: A developmental study of ethanol effect on behavior and physical dependence in mice. *Alcoholism Clin Exp Res* 1:325–333, 1977.

Zervoudakis, IA, Krauss, A, Fuchs, F: Infants of mothers treated with ethanol for premature labor. *Am J Obstet Gynecol* 137:713–718, 1980.

Appendix

Ten Question Drinking History

Beer:

How many times a week do you drink beer? _____

How many cans each time? _____

Ever drink more? _____

Wine:

How many times a week do you drink wine? _____

How many glasses each time? _____

Ever drink more? _____

Liquor:

How many times per week do you drink liquor? _____

How many drinks each time? _____

Ever drink more? _____

Has your drinking changed in the past year? _____

(Reprinted with permission from The American College of Obstetricians and Gynecologists, *Obstet Gynecol* 57(1):1–7, 1981.)

The Michigan Alcoholism Screening Test (MAST)

Directions: If a statement says something true about you, put a check (√) in the nearby space under YES. If a statement says something not true about you, put a check in the nearby space under NO. Please answer all the questions.

	YES	NO
1. Do you feel you are a normal drinker?		(2)
2. Have you ever awakened the morning after some drinking the night before and found that you could not remember a part of that evening?	(2)	
3. Does your wife/husband (or parents) ever worry or complain about your drinking?	(1)	
4. Can you stop drinking without a struggle after one or two drinks?		(2)
5. Do you ever feel bad about your drinking?	(1)	
6. Do friends or relatives think you are a normal drinker?		(2)
7. Do you ever try to limit your drinking to certain times of the day or to certain places?	(0)	
8. Are you always able to stop drinking when you want to?		(2)
9. Have you ever attended a meeting of Alcoholics Anonymous (AA)?	(5)	
10. Have you gotten into fights when drinking?	(1)	
11. Has drinking ever created problems with you and your wife/husband?	(2)	

	YES	NO

12. Has your wife/husband (or other family member) ever gone to anyone for help about your drinking? (2) ____

13. Have you ever lost friends (girlfriends or boyfriends) because of your drinking? (2) ____

14. Have you ever gotten into trouble at work because of your drinking? (2) ____

15. Have you ever lost a job because of your drinking? (2) ____

16. Have you ever neglected your obligations, your family or your work for two or more days in a row because you were drinking? (2) ____

17. Do you ever drink before noon? (1) ____

18. Have you ever been told you have liver trouble? (2) ____

19. Have you ever had delirium tremens (DTs), severe shaking, heard voices or seen things that weren't there after heavy drinking? (5) ____

20. Have you ever gone to anyone for help about your drinking? (5) ____

21. Have you ever been in a hospital because of your drinking? (5) ____

22. Have you ever been a patient in a psychiatric hospital or on a psychiatric ward of a general hospital where drinking was part of the problem? (2) ____

23. Have you ever been seen at a psychiatric or mental health clinic, or gone to a doctor, social worker, or clergyman for help with an emotional problem in which drinking played a part? (2) ____

24. Have you ever been arrested, even for a few hours, because of drunk behavior? (2) ____

	YES	NO
25. Have you ever been arrested for drunk driving or driving after drinking?	(2)	____

Total possible score = 54

If the patient scores 0–3 points, he/she is probably not alcoholic
4 points, borderline
5 or more, probable alcoholism

(Reprinted by permission, *Am J Psychiat* 127:1653–1658, 1971. © 1971, the American Psychiatric Association.)

The CAGE Questionnaire

	YES	NO
1. Have you ever felt you should <u>Cut down</u> on your drinking?	____	____
2. Have people <u>Annoyed</u> you by criticizing your drinking?	____	____
3. Have you ever felt bad or <u>Guilty</u> about your drinking?	____	____
4. Have you ever had a drink first thing in the morning to steady your nerves or get rid of a hang-over (<u>Eye-opener</u>)?	____	____

(If 2 or 3 out of 4 are answered yes, one should strongly suspect alcoholism.)

(Reprinted by permission, *Am J Psychiat* 131:1121–1123, 1974. © 1974, the American Psychiatric Association.)

Index